Quantitative
videoangiocardiography

Quantitative videoangiocardiography

R. P. VAN WIJK VAN BRIEVINGH

With a foreword by
prof. F. L. Meijler M.D.

Delft University Press/1975

ISBN 978-90-298-1700-4   ISBN 978-94-011-8075-7 (eBook)
DOI 10.1007/978-94-011-8075-7

To Joke, Matilde
and Arthur

*'Le coeur a ses raisons, que la raison ne connaît point;
on le sait en mille choses.'*

PASCAL, *Pensée 277*

Contents

Illustrations

Figures 2.2 and 4.1 are redrawn oscilloscope recordings.

The following illustrations have been reproduced from VAN WIJK VAN BRIEVINGH, (1974ᵃ) by courtesy of the European Journal of Cardiology (Excerpta Medica): 1.1; 2.8; 2.9; 2.10; 3.2; 3.4; 4.4; 4.5; 5.1(top); 6.2; 6.4.

Foreword

It is with great pleasure and gratitude that I fulfil the request to
write a foreword for this monograph.

In 1970 we asked the author to develop a system and construct the
equipment which would allow us to measure left ventricular end-diastolic and end-systolic volumes in patients with induced and autochtonous
arrhythmias. The question was evidently easier to ask than to answer,
as is demonstrated in and by this book. The complications which the
author encountered and had to overcome were numerous. He has indeed
shown great skill in solving most of the (bio-)technical problems, at
the same time showing an unheard- of organizational talent for lining
up the parts which together were to form the system which is described
in this book. One of the features of the system, the running videosubtraction, may in itself turn out to be of great importance for clinical cardiology. Apart from the pathophysiological significance of the
technique for left-ventricular volume measurement, its clinical relevance lies and should be looked for in the selection of patients for
cardiac and coronary bypass surgery and in the evaluation of the
results thereof.

This work is the fruit of a marriage between technology and medicine
and should be of equal interest, we hope, to medical engineers and
physicians, such as cardiologists and radiologists.

Preface

The study reported here has been carried out as a collaboration between
the Medical Engineering Group, Department of Electrical Engineering of
the Delft University of Technology and the Department of Cardiovascular
Diseases of the Utrecht University Hospital. The author feels it most
rewarding that a medical physicist has been willing to act as his pro-
motor and a cardiologist as his co-promotor, thus giving him the opportunity of learning a multidisciplinary field in the best situation
possible. The discussions with the co-referent prof.dr. D. Harting
contributed to a critical evaluation of theoretical and instrumental
aspects of the measurement system. The experience of participating in
the *in vivo* tests in the Laboratory for Experimental Cardiology with
dr. A.N.E. Zimmerman and in the catheterization laboratory with dr. T.
v.d. Werf and their staff has been a thorough initiation in the clinical
situation. The facilities granted by the Department of Electrical Engineering in a situation where the Medical Engineering Group still had to
find its proper place, are gratefully acknowledged. As the number of
co-authors of publications on the project shows, this thesis reports on
work done with members of both institutes; their enthousiastic contri-
bution has been one of my pleasures in this investigation.

Guiding the students who have participated in the project during their
4th year's- or M.Sc.E.E.-thesis subjects has been a most satisfying
aspect of my daily work.

The Dutch Foundation for Fundamental Medical Research, FUNGO, has granted a subsidy for this project, thus making it possible to apply advanced
technology to the solution of the clinical problem posed.

Quantitative
videoangiocardiography

I. INTRODUCTION

1. Medical Background

The action of the heart as a muscular pump cannot be defined completely
without knowledge of its change in shape and volume from instant to
instant throughout the cardiac cycle. The changes in dimensions of the
left ventricle, correlated with its functional changes will provide a
more complete understanding of its performance (SOLOFF,1966)[†]. Results,
obtained from measurements on isolated myocardial preparations, cannot
be extrapolated without reserve to the function of the intact ventricle
because of its heterogeneous contractile performance (FISHER,1967;
SONNENBLICK,1974). The use of anaesthetized open chest animal preparations for the study of ventricular dimensions is of limited value, as
no clear relationship between these measurements and those actually
occurring in the awake intact animal and man can be made (HAWTHORNE,1967).
Furthering our understanding of myocardial performance depends among
others on the assessment of the absolute accuracy of available methods
of measuring left ventricular volume throughout the cardiac cycle
(DAVILA,1966[a]).

   The first to measure the volume of the left ventricular cavity (LVV)
was STEPHEN HALES in 1733. He determined the water displacement of

---

[†]For short, each reference is quoted by the name of the first author
only. Internal reports are collected in a separate list.

bees'wax casts and calculated cardiac output by multiplying this volume
by the normal pulse rate of the subject (horses, oxen, sheep, dogs and
man). In 1844, KUERSCHNER still supported the view that the ventricles
expelled completely the blood volume they contained. He based himself
on observations in chickens, slaughtered animals and autopsies on human
corpses. At that time, however, the equal capacity of the left and
right ventricle during life is already indicated. HIFFELSHEIM and ROBIN
published in 1864 the results of an extensive investigation in which
the volumes of wax casts of left and right atria and ventricles were
compared. It was concluded beyond any doubt that in rabbits, dogs as
well as in humans the volume of the left and right ventricles was
20-30% larger than that of the corresponding atria. In adults an LVV
of 143-212 ml is reported, whereas the left atrial volume amounts to
100-130 ml. Corrections of 10-15 ml for the right ventricular volume
and 12-17 ml for the LVV were taken into consideration because of
papillary muscles and *chordae tendinae*. The consequences of these findings were considered crucial in the explanation of cardiac function:

> *"Ces comparaisons établies d'après des mesures de capacité
> réelle, sont à divers points de vue utiles pour l'étude de la
> physiologie du coeur et du poumon, contrairement à l'opinion
> de ceux qui les considéraient comme devant sans intérêt, lors
> même qu'elles viendraient à être faites. Leur importance
> repose particulièrement sur cette conséquence: si l'oreillette
> ne peut pas remplir le ventricule, sa systole ne saurait être
> ce que l'on a cru. Elle n'a pas l'énergie, la puissance subite
> qu'on lui prête. Elle se désemplit comme un réservoir servant
> à approvisionner le ventricule. Cette considération puisée
> dans les faits sans réplique, ôte aux oreillettes le rôle de
> centre circulatoire principal que leur attribuaient quelques
> savants au détriment des ventricules."*

Furthermore, the exact measurement of heart-cavity volumes is used by
Robin,(1864) to square accounts with older views held on changes in the
volume and nature of the blood itself:

> *"Aujourd'hui, en suivant l'ordre d'idées qui occupait HELVETIUS
> (1864), on ne songerait plus à une condensation imaginaire du
> sang, mais à la diminution de volume qu'il éprouve en passant
> au travers du poumon, où il laisse échapper de la vapeur
> d'eau."* (ROBIN,1864).

The concept that the maximum LVV equals the volume of blood pumped out was retained until in '888 ROY and ADAMI introduced the residual ventricular volume into the discussion of cardiac dynamics. Thus stroke volume (SV) had to be understood to be the difference of end-diastolic volume (EDV) and end-systolic volume (ESV), the values of LVV at the beginning of ventricular concentration and the opening of the aortic valves respectively. They made observations in open-chest dogs by feeling with the little finger via an incision into the apex. This method supported measurements on the amount of residual blood in the ventricle:

> *"It is generally asserted that, at the end of each contraction, the ventricle is always empty of blood, a view which is evidently opposed to what we have just said as to varying amount of residual blood in the ventricles at the end of systole. The following experiment, even were there no other evidence at hand, conclusively shows, we think, that generally received views upon this subject are erroneous.*
> *. . . it can be felt that, in each contraction, the lower part of the ventricular cavity closes completely, the musculi papillares coming into contact with one another; the upper part of the cavity, however, lying between the valves and the papillary muscles does not become emptied".*

A description of the pumping function may be given in two different sets of terms. Myocardial properties and ventricle dimensions together with the pressure in the ventricular cavity determine the ventricle's performance. The latter can be expressed either in terms of muscle variables such as stress and strain in the muscular shell, or in hydraulic variables as the volume and velocity of the ejected blood (SANDLER, 1969). As the second set of quantities can be measured in the intact subject, whereas the first cannot, myocardial muscle properties can only be deduced to the extent they are reflected in secondary quantities. In 1895, FRANK observed that the systolic intraventricular pressure of the isolated frog's heart rose with increased filling, whereby the force of contraction became greater with the muscular fiber length. This performance of the ventricle was described by STARLING (1918):

> *" The energy of contraction, however measured, is a function of the length of the muscle fibre."*

Nowadays it is understood that the heart's pumping function is under control of many factors, of which the purely contractile aspects can

be analysed seperately in the isolated perfused heart (MEIJLER,1969),
or the isolated papillary muscle (BRUTSAERT,1969). As the organ under
these circumstances is not subject to nervous or chemical influences
originating outside of it, intrinsic readjustments to varying conditions, *i.e.* autoregulation, may be studied. SARNOFF (1960;1962)
distinguishes heterometric autoregulation which occurs on a beat-to-beat
basis from homeometric autoregulation which requires at least a few
beats to develop fully. The second kind tends to keep end-diastolic
pressure and fiber length constant after an initial increase in activity,
which is achieved by an increase of "myocardial contractility" (BRUTSAERT,
1973). Quantitative description of this most important "non-quantity" is
already very difficult in isolated papillary muscle (NOBLE,1974). An
analysis of the performance of the intact ventricle as defined by stroke
volume or stroke work (SW) by BRAUNWALD, ROSS and SONNENBLICK (1967)
leads to three factors. The *preload* defined by the EDV, reflects the
initial fiber lengths or tensions in the myocardium. The *afterload,*
defined by the end-diastolic aortic pressure against which the left ventricle has to pump out the blood, reflects the force to be developed by
the individual fibers. The third factor, called the *contractile state of
the myocardium* reflects the fibers' force-velocity-length relations, but
is not definable by one single physical quantity. Because of the intricate architecture of the ventricular wall, which is composed of several
layers of muscular fibers with different orientation (RUSHMER,1951[a]),
a translation of fiber characteristics into hydraulic parameters is difficult. The maximum relative rate of change of the intraventricular
pressure $\left[(dP/dt)/P\right]_{max}$ is a frequently used measure. BOOM (1973) arguments that the dP/dt *vs* P slope provide a better index for myocardial
contractility. From a survey by PETERSON (1974), however, it appears
that contractility indices computed from LV-angiographic data are to be
preferred to those derived from pressure alone. By its shape, the
pressure-volume diagram is indicative for the pumping function of the
left ventricle. The area enclosed by the loop is a measure for the
external work, SW, supplied by the ventricular muscle (DODGE,1962;
BAUEREISEN,1964; BUNNELL,1965). The time-varying pressure-volume ratio of

4

the ventricle has been shown by SUGA (1974) to be linked to the contractile state of the heart in the excised, supported canine left ventricle. By means of a thin-walled or a finite-element model, stress and strain distribuations in the LV-wall can be computed from its dimensions as determined from angiography, together with the intracavitary pressure (GHISTA,1969; HOOD,1969; JANZ,1972). Besides several clinical applications for LVV-measurement results as mentioned by DODGE (1966), these may also be utilized for parametric simulation of the left ventricular control mechanism (GHISTA,1966; DODGE,1966)

Another form of modeling is becoming of medical interest as a method for supporting the clinician's judgement. The use of computer graphics allows the construction and real-time or slow-motion display of pseudo-threedimensional pictures of the LV-cavity from angiographic contour data and an assumed geometry (COULAM,1972; GREENLEAF,1972; SANDLER,1972, HEINTZEN,1974[b]). These presentations, which can be rotated so that they may be viewed from different perspectives, give the opportunity to apply mental as well as mathematical identification processes to correlate various surface forms with various heart functions. It should be borne in mind, however, that no model can give better results than the underlying assumptions allow. In the case of this "morphometry" method, one of the limiting factors is that a set of ventricular casts is not available, which is representative for various contraction phases in normals and patients.

As an extension of the study of RR-interval-contractility relationships during random stimulation of the isolated heart (MEIJLER,1968), dependence of stroke volume and stroke work in the intact ventricle upon the duration of preceding RR-intervals is a major part of the investigations at the Utrecht University Department of Cardiovascular Diseases. In order to separate the preload and afterload effects, the EDV and systolic aortic pressure have to be measured together with the ESV and ventricular pressure. A quantitative analysis of LV-pumping function in coronary patients is furthermore of utmost importance for giving an indication for coronary surgery and for judgement of the results thereof. Determination of contractile indices at rest is often unsatisfactory because of considerable overlap between patients with and without heart disease. A better insight into the actual myocardial contractility of an individual patient might be provided by analyzing the response of the left ventricle to additional loading. The latter should be chosen such, that peripherally located compensatory mechanisms do not interfere. This is the case if artificial stimulation of the ventricle is performed in such a way, that a suitable sequence of RR-intervals occurs. The response in parameters describing LV-function in that case is solely determined by the ventricle's compensatory action as peripheral effects do not have time to develop.

Because of the sientific and clinical relevance of a method in which myocardial contractility may be studied on the basis of relatively simple electric pacing in a well-chosen rhythm, the development of a rather intricate system for measuring the ventricle's response seems justified. There exists no complete theory for describing the very complex nature of cardiac control, so it is of great importance to gather simultaneously as much information as possible.

We expect that the method described in this thesis will increase the amount of relevant data without an extra burden to the patient.

2. *Review of Possible Methods*

The relationship between diastolic size and systolic discharge of the left ventricle of cats and monkeys has, due to the war, been assessed only in 1955 from an X-ray motion picture originally made in 1944 to demonstrate the effect of centrifugal forces on the circulation, (GAUER, 1955). The configuration of the heart chambers and the mechanics of ventricular contraction have been studied extensively in dogs by cine-fluorography. Additional information was gained by implanted marker experiments leading to a better understanding of the functional anatomy of ventricular contraction (RUSHMER,1951[a],1951[b],1953). Many sophisticated engineering techniques have been applied to study the dynamic geometry of the left ventricle. Dimensional data from implanted transducers in combination with pressure and flow measurements in the experimental animal have provided more insight in left-ventricular function. The first measurement of LVV from biplane X-ray studies in man was reported in 1956 (DODGE). In 1966, 1967 and 1968 symposia have been devoted to the problem of measuring left ventricular volume (DAVILA,1966[a];DODGE,1967; HAWTHORNE,1969). A detailed summary of the work on dimensional analysis of the heart in the nineteen-sixties has been given by SANDLER (1970).

Besides by direct measurement of internal or external dimensions of the LV, the pump function of the heart is also studied with indicator dilution methods (TEN HOOR,1969). Agents used as an indicator are: hypertonic NaCl-solution (HOLT,1957), optical dye, *e.g.* indocyanine green (FOX,1960; TEN HOOR,1967), saline "thermodilution" (THORPE,1960; VAN DER WERF,1965), radioactive nuclides (DONATO,1962[a],1962[b]) or radio-paque material (WOOD,1964; RUTISHAUER,1969; HEINTZEN,1971[a]; BUERSCH,1972). Systematic differences between results of indicator dilution and angiographic methods for determining LVV as apparent in the literature have been analyzed by HALLERMAN (1965), who has arrived at the conclusion that the EDV as calculated by the dilution method is systematically over-estimated by a factor 2 due to incomplete mixing of the indicator. Thus the angiographic method is thought to be the more reliable of the two. In the future sono-cardiography may prove to be a clinically useful method especially in children because of its non-evasive nature (BOM, 1972). It has already been shown that LVV, as measured by ultrasound, even when calculated by simple geometric model from internal LV diameters gives good correlation with angiographically determined values over a wide range of ESV and EDV (CRAIGE,1972). Determination of LVV from mono- or biplane angiograms, however, is at present considered the standard method. It has been chosen as the basis of the system developed by us.

3. Aspects of the Method Chosen

"Quantitative Videoangiocardiography" is a measuring technique in which dimensions of heart cavities--mostly the left ventricle--, marked with radiopaque medium, are derived from their X-ray projections as represented by video-signals. The less descriptive term "Videometry" is also used for this technique. The basic information is given by the temporal changes of spatial density gradients (HEINTZEN,1972). The scanning principle of the television system converts these into an electric signal, sampling the picture each frame. During the past two decades, video techniques have found increasing application in investigations of the cardiovascular system (GLANCY,1973). Electronic manipulation of the videosignal is a relatively easy way of changing the picture's properties. Linear operations (changing the frequency spectrum) as well as non-linear ones (amplitude-dependent amplification) may be used (PIKE, 1962). These techniques have been shown to improve diagnostic accuracy (REVESZ, 1969). Furthermore, subtraction of a picture without added contrast from one of the same structure after contrast medium injection, may be performed electronically (GROH,1967) to yield a picture with less disturbing details. A trained human observer can then draw the LV-outlines with a monitor-lightpen system. The contours are available as pulses in the videosignal with reference to the synchronization pattern and may thus be easily interfaced to a computer (ALDERMAN,1973). Finally, as not the whole TV-frame is needed for determining of the LV-outline, storing of other synchronous physiological information on parts of the same data carrier is an attractive possibility (OSYPKA,1971), which may lead to data recording on one medium with the high information density inherent to magnetic material.

The set-up has been chosen on the basis of an analysis of requirements, of which the results can be stated as follows:

A biplane X-ray installation, designed to obtain pictures which are interpreted visually, has to be calibrated as it will be part of a measurement system.

The contrast medium has to be injected in fractions at selected moments of the cardiac cycle. With a given maximum amount of medium, the number of fractions has to be as large as is still consistent with the detectability of the LV-border.

All pertinent information has to be recorded on one medium so as to preserve time relationships and patient identification. Coding of data into the videosignal representing the image information has been chosen as the most flexible method.

Videosignals representing the X-ray shadow should be preprocessed (videosubtraction, contrast enhancement) thus facilitating contour detection.

Determination of the LV-contour has to be based on density information as well as on a-priori knowledge of the cardiologically trained observer. Thus a semi-automatical system is chosen with regard to the accuracy of measurement required.

The conversion of contour- and other data has to be chosen in such a way, that computer handling is possible.

For calculation of the LVV, a geometric model must be used which is related as closely as possible to the anatomic reality. The position of the ventricle relative to the coordinate system has to be taken into account too.

The software package also must comprise calculations with the data measured, e.g. PV-loop, SW, correlation with RR-intervals. Preliminary reports of the measurement procedure have been published (VAN WIJK VAN BRIEVINGH,1973[a],1974[a]) the various aspects will be elaborated in the following chapters.

4. Set-up of the Measurement System

As shown in Fig. 1.1, the measurement system makes use of the catheterization room equipped with a biplane X-ray installation, inclusive the coordination room as well as the computer system already present at the Utrecht University Department of Cardiovascular Diseases. To convert the X-ray installation into a part of the measurement system, special features had to be added. Equipment for data registration and evaluation has been built at the Medical Engineering Group, Department of Electrical Engineering, of the Delft University of Technology. For the evaluation phase of the measurement process a special room has been equipped.

The registration part of the measurement system comprises a biplane X-ray installation, synchronization and timing circuits, coding devices and a videodisk. At certain moments in the cardiac cycle, a quantum of contrast medium is administered followed by X-ray flashes, controlled by a time programming unit using a microcomputer. Shadow projections of the left ventricle on the image intensifier screens are converted into visible light pictures, viewed by television cameras. The video-signals representing the middle parts of the two orthogonal projections are combined in a new videoframe to which coded extra measurement information is also added by the so-called Vidicor, Anacor and Digicor, to be described in Chapter V.

The evaluation part consists of a light-pen system, a digital contour memory inclusive video-computer interface, decoding devices and a DIGITAL EQUIPMENT PDP-15 computer. Image correction, contrast expansion and other types of filtering as well as subtraction may be performed readily on the electric signal representing the X-ray images. A trained human observer determines the contours of the LV shadows from the picture on a monitor. These contours are fed to the computer by means of an interface. From the contour data, measurement parameters as introduced separately and a geometric model which describes the form of the LV-cavity, the LV-volume is calculated.

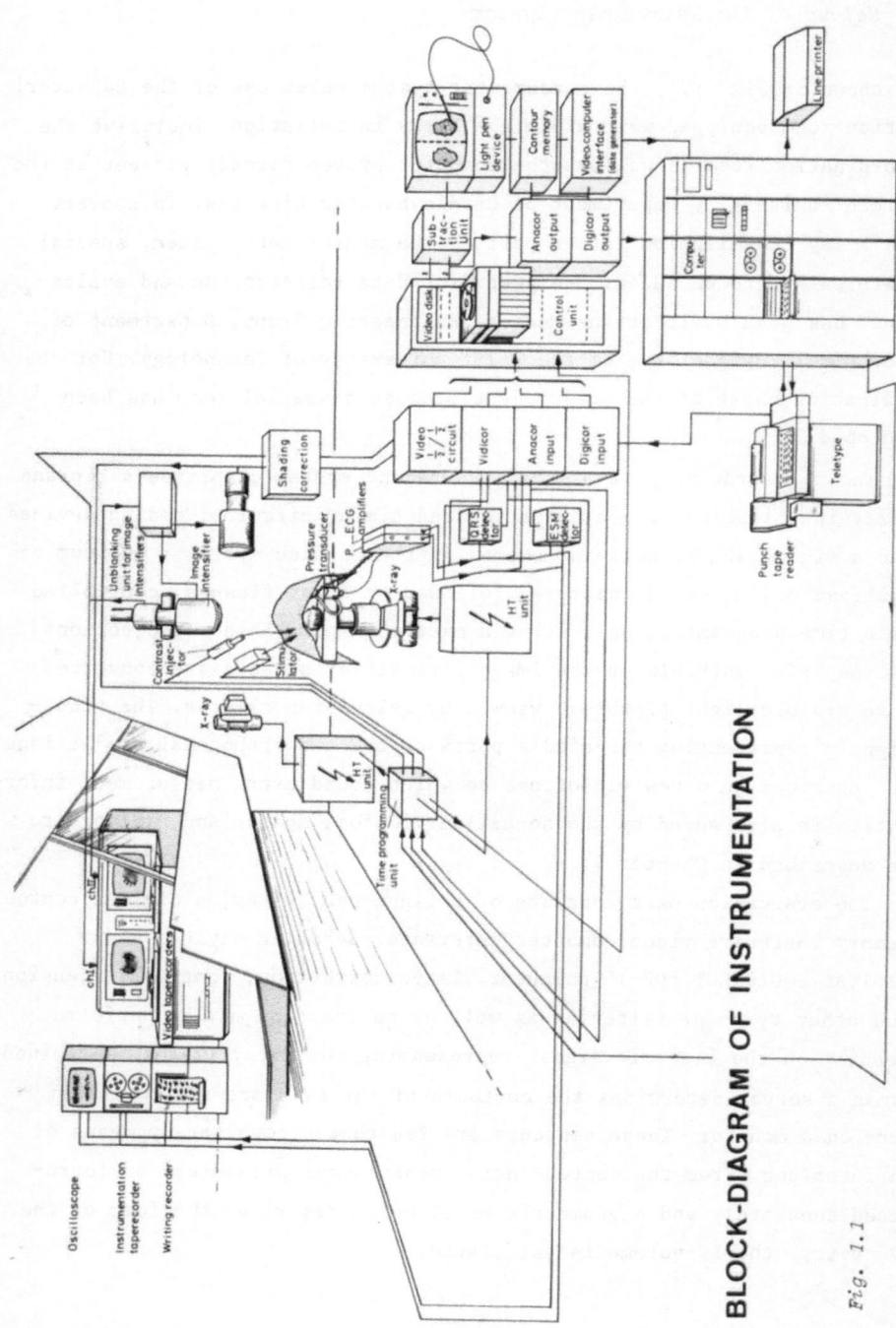

BLOCK-DIAGRAM OF INSTRUMENTATION

Fig. 1.1

12

II. THE X-RAY INSTALLATION AS A PART OF THE MEASUREMENT SYSTEM

1. *Introduction*

New techniques for the investigation of size and position of intracorporal organs without disturbance of the anatomic integrity of the subject became possible after the discovery of X-rays by ROENTGEN (1895). Only two years later, attempts were made to record the movements of internal organs by application of moving picture techniques, which by then were barely one decade old (MACINTYRE,1897). A method by which it was possible to record the image of the heart, free from distortion, from the fluoroscopic screen was described by MORITZ in 1900. The position of a vertically collimated X-ray beam was recorded on a drawing table by means of a mechanical construction which could be moved with respect to the patient. By moving the X-ray tube along the heart shadow's border, a point-by-point registration of the undistorted heart contour was obtained (orthodiagraphy).
A different method for correction of the distortion due to the divergence of the X-ray beam, making use of the measured shift of the image if a known displacement is given to the tube, was described by BARDEEN in 1918, who used a teleradiographic installation (tube-screen distance 2 meters).

The adaptation of moving picture methods to investigate specifically the motions of the heart was described by EYKMAN in 1909. Two years later, LOMAN and COMANDON (1911) invented indirect cineroentgenography, in which a fluoroscopic screen is photographed, rather than having X-rays directly striking the film. The latter method was described first by GROEDEL (1909), who obtained four pictures per second by an exposure time of 1/20 sec. with a primitive film changer of 24 cassettes coupled to a rotating lead disk with a window in it, placed between the patient and the X-ray tube. The forerunner of the modern roll film changer has been developed by RUGGELS and FLEISCHER (1925), and was used by CHAMBERLAIN and DOCK (1926) to study the different phases of heart motion.

A further improvement of the accuracy of total heart volume calculation from roentgenograms became possible by the development of horizontal and transversal tomography during recent years, based on the work of ZIEDSES DES PLANTES (1934). By opposite synchronous rotation of the X-ray tube and the film cassette around two vertical axes while the subject is stationary, only the points in the plane which is cut by the X-ray beam through the subject are depicted sharply, while the shadows of all other structures are smeared out. So the pictures of slices through the subject can be obtained, and used to compose the cardiac ED-volume; (BROUSTET, 1953, 1955, 1960, 1961; DUHAMEL, 1954; BRAUN, 1960). GEBHARDT (1957) described the use of simultaneous planigraphy in seven parallel planes for this purpose. The effects of various factors as projection and body position on the roentgenological determination of cardiac volume have also been described in literature (LARSSON, 1948; KJELLBERG, 1951; KOENIG, 1967; BERGSTRØM, 1969[a], 1969[b]).
The total cardiac volume and the transverse diameter of the heart silhouette have been brought in relation with the body surface area as computed from weight and height by JONSELL (1939) and UNGERLEIDER (1939), a method which is used nowadays to compute a volume index from the EDV (YANG, 1972).

Next to the determination of the volume of the whole cardiac structure from roentgenograms, measurement of intracardiac volumes became possible after introduction of the angiographic method in cardiovascular radiology (TIMM, 1947). Use of the radiopaque dye as a dilution indicator has been introduced by SINCLAIR (1960) and WOOD (1962), and turned into an accepted method (RUTISHAUSER, 1969; HEINTZEN, 1971[a]; BUERSCH, 1972; HEUCK, 1973). Thus, the X-ray installation has become a measurement tool for densitometric as well as for morphologic purposes.

Introduction of image intensifiers (HOLST, 1934; COLTMAN, 1948; MORGAN, 1951; TEVES, 1952) and television systems (BISCHOFF, 1961) into radiology has reduced patient dose and improved image quality considerably (MOSELEY, 1965, 1969; STIEVE, 1966[a]; HERSTEL, 1968). Modern television methods have also given the possibility of contour movement determination, called videokymography, radarkymography or video-tracking (LINDBERG, 1972; GLANCY, 1973; KAZAMIAS, 1973; LEVITSKY, 1973).

2. *Central synchronization of the X-ray/television system*

After the introduction of image intensifiers, the most important recent
improvement of diagnostic radiology has been pulsed X-ray radiation
(BISCHOFF, 1962). The use of X-ray flashes, triggered by the action of
a sphygmograph, was described as early as 1902 (EYKMAN, 1909). Because
of the short exposure times thus obtained, blurring of pictures due to
movements of the subject is greatly diminished and the dose administered to the patient is reduced in comparison with fluoroscopy (PENN,
1967). In cinematography, the blurring if present is due to movement
and in correspondance with the pulse duration. The film exposure time
however, is longer than the pulse duration, because of the image intensifier screens' decay time. During the pulse, the intensity as well as
the quality (energy spectrum) of the radiation vary, so data on the
integrated brightness produced as a function of tube voltage (kV) and
tube current (mA)--which are in general not available from the manu-
facturer--have to be used in exposure calculations (HEINTZEN, 1971[f]),
and (video-)densitometry (HEINTZEN, 1971[i]; MOLDENHAUER, 1972).

A second problem occurring in pulsed X-ray installations is posed by
the imperfect smoothing and/or regulation in the high tension generator.
The influence of the ripple voltage and loading effects is not negligi-
ble as the radiation dose rate at the input screen grows with a power
of the tube voltage, the exponent of which is quoted to be 4 to 5
(SPIEGLER, 1957) or 3 to 4 (SEEMAN, 1968). The fact that this exponent
is higher than the number 2 encountered in an unattenuated X-ray beam
can be explained by a diminishing absorption within the subject, and a
higher efficiency of the sensitive screen at higher energies (CSORBA,
1971). The effect of the high tension variation due to the ripple voltage on the tube is that of a flickering image at the output phosphor
of the image intensifier, because of interference of the radiation
pulse period and that of the high voltage ripple (PENN, 1967; HEINTZEN,
1969, 1971[f]). This interference will not occur if these periods are
equal to or differ a whole number with the ripple period. The last case
is only true if the rectifiers in the HT-generator have equal conduc-

tance; otherwise the three phases of the voltage will have different
amplitude. In videosystems, the required isochronism is relatively easy
to obtain, as the master oscillator of the synchronization pulse generator may be phase-locked to the mains, and the X-ray flashes are given
at moments which bear constant relationship to the vertical synchronization pulses. The X-ray radiation is administered in pulses of 1 to 2
milliseconds wide. The target of the plumbicon camera tube acts as a
short-term memory (retention time about 30 ms) so that if the X-ray
image is formed during the vertical synchronization pulse, it may be
scanned in the interval between pulses.

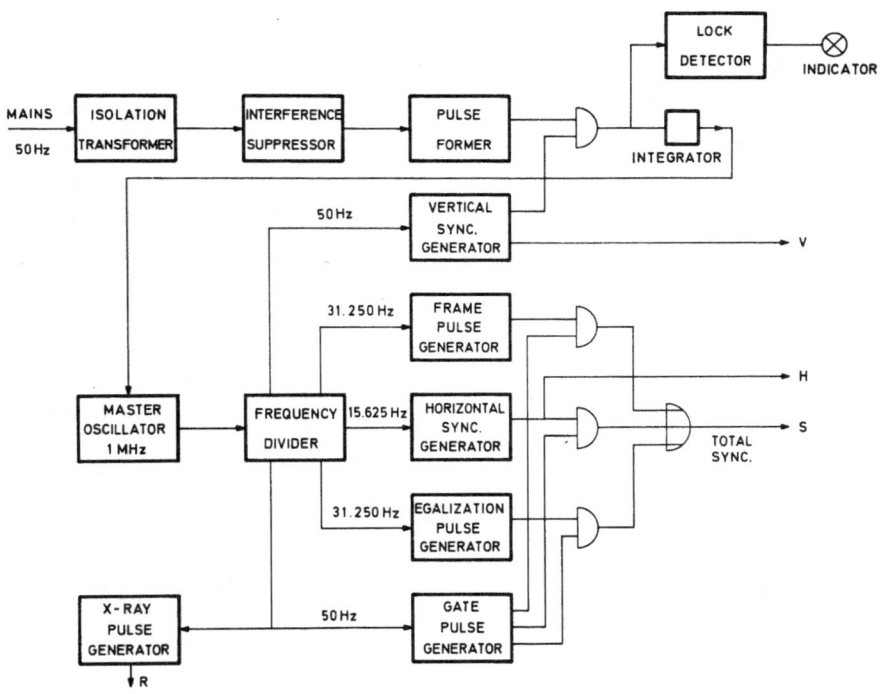

Fig. 2.1 Central Synchronization

By proper adjustment of the phase, the X-ray pulse can be triggered at the moment one of the rectifiers is in the conducting state. Then the internal resistance of the HT-generator is lowest, and the loading effect minimal. The central synchronization unit is shown in Fig.2-1. The phase reference is derived from the mains, and compared with the 50 Hz vertical synchronization pulse obtained from a master oscillator. The latter is controlled by the integrated difference. This phase-locked loop has been designed according to the stability requirements of the video disc (plus or minus 5.10^{-4} per ms) as the long-term stability of the mains frequency is better than 2.10^{-4} per day, but may have short-term variations of plus or minus 2.10^{-3}. In this way, also the occurrence of a dark bar on the video screen caused by interference between the vertical synchronization pulse period and the radiation pulses is eliminated (HEINTZEN, 1971[g]). The effect of electronic gating of the image intensifiers to diminish the influence of the scattering from the alternating X-ray source in a biplane installation is described in the article quoted as well as by DUEMMLING (1969[a]). In our installation this unblanking facility could not be provided by the manufacturer. Fig. 2.2. shows the influence discussed.

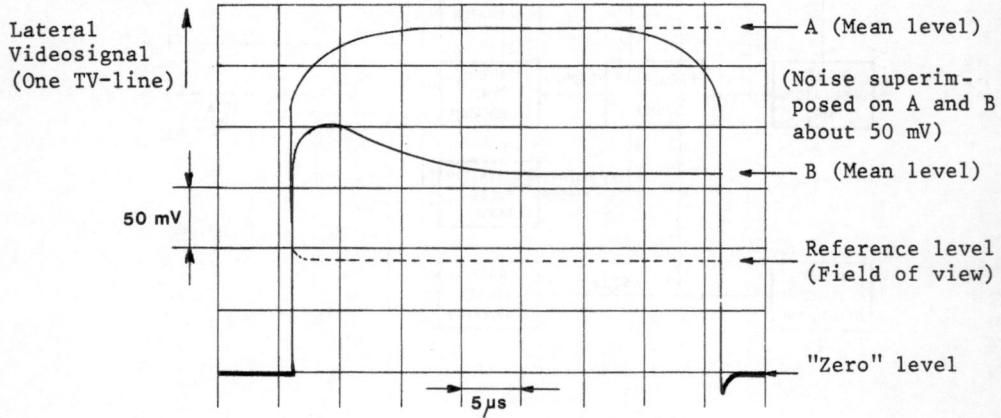

A: Lateral X-rays, 60 kV, tube current control switched on.
B: Without lateral X-rays, with frontal X-rays, 90 kV, tube current control switched on. Scattering medium: 25 cm water absorber.

Fig. 2.2 Effect of Scattered Radiation (Biplane)

Coupling of the X-ray pulse frequency to the 50 or 25 Hz (corresponding to television frames and fields respectively) of the videosystem means a fixed sampling frequency which naturally does not harmonize with the heart rate. Therefore, artificial stimulation of the patient's heart is required as will be demonstrated in Chapter III, ssection 4. According to JONSELL (1939), triggering of the X-ray source--by means of the exposure relay--from the ECG was used as early as 1939 in making biplane still pictures at certain moments in the cardiac cycle. The reduction of the radiation dose administered to the patient as made possible by the image-intensifier/videosystem combination may also be exploited in fluoroscopy. The clinician needs some time to interpret the picture; it seems unreasonable to irradiate the patient during this period. The introduction of the videodisk into the clinic gives the opportunity of repeated presentation of only one stored television image obtained by pulsed fluoroscopy (BAKER, 1967). Dependent on the type of problem, a reduction of the dose to the patient of 90% (DORPH, 1970) or 2 to 60 times (GROLLMAN, 1972) has been reported.

3. Imaging Characteristics of the Image-intensifier/Television System

The methods one can use to extract quantitative data from radiographs are dependent upon those qualities of the image which lend themselves to analysis (ROCKOFF,1972). Attempts to measure image quality in radiology (STIEVE,1966) as well as the use of techniques from linear systems theory (PFEILER,1968) have been described. The latter stem from the application in optics as summarized by THOMPSON (1970), the theory of "FOURIER optics" is well established (GOODMAN,1968). The historical development of the optical transfer function (OTF) has been sketched by BAKER, (1970). In the assessment of radiologic imaging, besides the resolution, quantified in terms of the optical transfer function, the contrast range, defined as the maximal contrast difference present, is to be taken into consideration as a distinct criterion. At a given dose, both may be expressed in a single criterion of system performance, the "information capacity" (GREGG,1966). From this quantity (about 2 bits.mm^{-2} at 0,1 mR exposure rate at the entrance window for a 9" image intensifier + TV chain), the bandwidth of the TV chain is to be calculated. The concept "metric information capacity of an image" had been used for this purpose by BOUWERS in 1958 already (BOUWERS,1962) and is utilized by FRIEDELL (1965), to determine a "ratio of information index to patient dose". Relations between information capacity and object spectrum in radiographic images have been established by KANAMORI (1970). Many aspects of image reproduction by a line raster process have been discussed by several authors in BIBERMAN (1973).

In transmitting a moving image, the relation between the input and output modulations of the image transfer system depends on one temporal and two spatial coordinates. The corresponding three-dimensional FOURIER spectra presenting one temporal and two spatial frequencies determine the complex OTF of the system, which may be considered linear in practice, if only small contrasts are present in the image. These contrasts define the modulation $(I_2-I_1)/(I_2+I_1)$ of intensity in adjacent points 1 and 2. Consideration of non-linearity in image transfer systems has been described by SAYANAGI (1969). If isotropy and isoplanasy may be assumed,

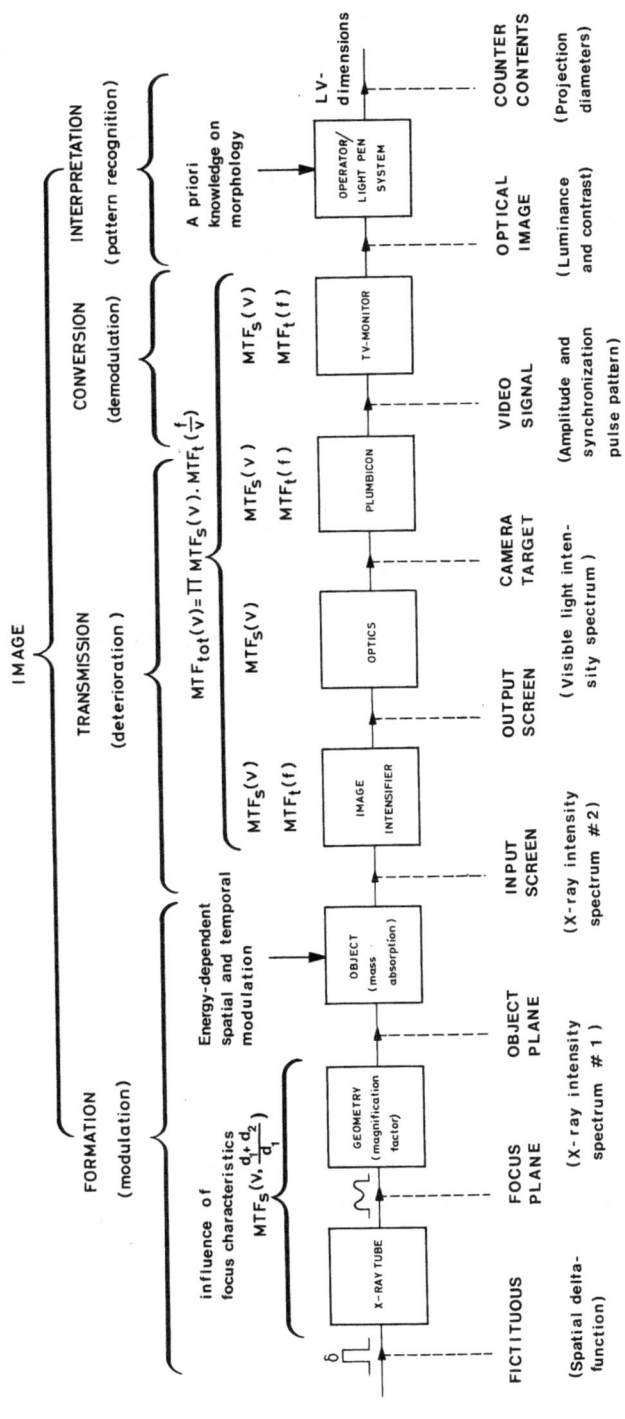

BLOCK DIAGRAM OF X-RAY/TV-SYSTEM

Fig. 2.3

21

which is at least the case within limited regions, "patches", of the image plane, the spatial behaviour can be described in one dimension. This means that the transfer properties are unaffected by the spatial directions, and constant over the part of the image plane considered. Size and shape of the patches have to be established from the experiment. Furthermore, from the design of the transmission system components it appears that the temporal behaviour of the system is independent of the spatial characteristics. So, the total OTF is the combined result of an OTF_t and an OTF_s. In practice, mostly only the moduli of these complex functions are used, which are called modulation transfer functions, $MTF_t(f)$ and $MTF_s(\nu)$, of which the latter is defined by the International Commission on Optics as the normalized modulus of the FOURIER transform of the line spread function. The overall MTF of an image transmission system may be found from the MTF's of its components by multiplication (SCHOTT, 1966).

The block diagram of the imaging system is shown in Fig. 2.3., where, the image is described as generated by a modulation process, transmitted by the image-intensifier/television system, and after demodulation interpreted by a human observer to obtain the left ventricular shadow contours. The imperfections of the "carrier", the X-ray beam, which are mainly caused by the finite dimensions and anisotropic intensity distribution of the focal spot, have to be taken into account also, as they do affect the resulting image (GROH, 1973). The latter is formed by mass absorption of the X-ray beam; in angiography the added contrast medium is the important factor in this process. In this modulation process, the geometrical unsharpness (penumbra width) caused by the finite focal spot dimensions may also be described by means of an MTF. LUBBERS (1967) derived and experimentally verified the following expression for it in the case of a completely radiopaque, plane-parallel plate with its edge at the beam centre, irradiated perpendicularly by a uniformly radiating rectangular focus of width a, the focal-spot-object distance and object-film distance being d_1 and d_2 respectively:

$$MTF_s(\nu) = \left| \frac{\sin \pi \nu ad_2/d_1}{\pi \nu ad_2/d_1} \right| \quad \ldots \ldots \ldots \ldots \ldots \ldots \quad (2.1)$$

RAO (1968) took also the shape of the focus into account, by investigating the MTF with the angles of projection of the focal spot. The MTF-curves obtained with the measuring slit parallel to the line focus exhibited maximal attenuation. The same author (RAO,1973) showed that the MTF of an imaging system is affected adversely when the geometrical magnification factor, $(d_1+d_2)/d_1$, increases. In our measurement of total MTF to be described, the effect mentioned will be automatically included as these are performed with the complete X-ray installation as it is used in practice.

The dynamic unsharpness, described quantitavely by the temporal modulation transfer function, MTF_t, is of importance in our system, as the ventricular wall to be observed may reach speeds of about 100 mm.s^{-1}. The MTF_t varies considerably with the exposure rate at the image intensifier entrance window (HERSTEL, 1968). In the case of a moving object, the velocity component, v, of the structure observed parallel to the image plane and the spatial frequency component of interest, ν, determine a temporal frequency, f, for which the $MTF_t(f)$ gives the corresponding unsharpness. The temporal resolution is mainly determined by the persistence time of the image intensifier screens which amounts to an average value of 2,6 ms (DUEMMLING,1972) and by the TV-camera tube (FRANKEN,1972 ; RITMAN,1973). In the case of pulsed radiation, the temporal resolution is practically determined by the pulse duration, τ, according to:

$$MTF_t(f) = \left| \frac{\sin \pi f \tau}{\pi f \tau} \right| = \left| \frac{\sin \pi \nu v f}{\pi \nu v f} \right| \quad \ldots \ldots \ldots \ldots \quad (2.2)$$

If continuous radiation had been used, the reciprocal of the frame rate should be substituted for τ in this formula, being the integration time per frame. As the pulse duration is of the order of 2 ms and the frame duration amounts to 20 ms, a pulsed X-ray-television system is able to record movements faster than corresponds with the frame rate. The sampling frequency of the system, however, is equal to the frame rate, and should be sufficient for the dynamic processes under study.

In order to use the biplane X-ray installation at the clinic as a part of a measurement system, its spatial and temporal resolution had to be measured. For this purpose, stationary and moving test objects, mostly slits, have been described (HERSTEL,1968; DUEMMLING,1969). If we determine the disappearance frequently in the object plane, ν_c, than with the known magnification factor, also an effective focal spot size, EFS, may be determined according to HOLLANDER (1972):

$$EFS = \frac{d_1 + d_2}{\nu_c d_2} \quad \cdots \cdots \cdots \cdots \cdots \cdots \cdots \cdots \cdots \cdots \quad (2.3)$$

A method, making use of the definition of MTF_s, has been described by TIMMER,(1973), and was used by us (Internal Report M121)[')]. The OTFs of the total system, comprising focal spot, magnification factor, and television system with the registration part included, but exclusive the monitor, is determined by FOURIER transformation of a measured line spread function. The latter was found as the system response on the absorption of a gold wire of 200 μm diameter, placed at the position corresponding with the patient's heart, under normal conditions of X-ray tube voltage and current, so as to reproduce the focal spot size. Although this measurement poses severe noise problems, the BUCKY-filters, normally present to reduce scattered radiation (HONDIUS BOLDINGH,1964), have been removed in order to obviate the anisotropy effect caused by the parallel lead septa. After sampling and averaging of the relevant part of the videosignal, the response was digitized and the FOURIER

───────────────

[')] Thanks are due to F. Timmer, Image Quality Group, Medical Systems Division SAII-4, N.V. Philips' Gloeilampenfabrieken, Eindhoven

24

transform calculated. In order to correct for the low-frequency drop in
this curve caused by the limited width of the response due to noise
limitations, the edge response was measured as well, giving the low-
frequency part of the MTF_s-curve including the 100% value. The test object used is given in Fig. 2.4.[')], the responses and the OTF in Fig. 2.5.

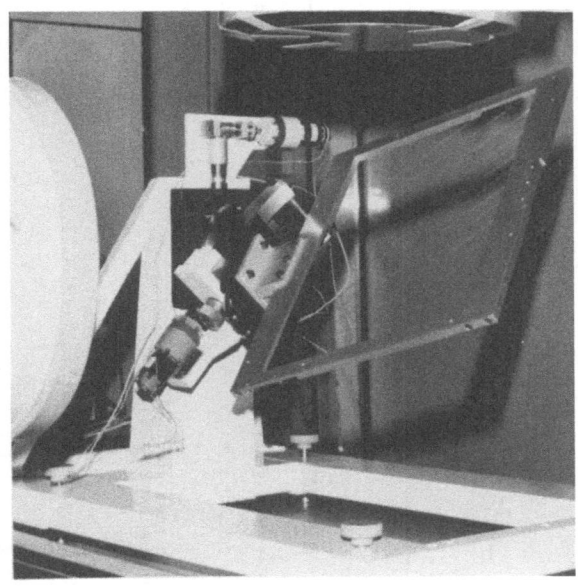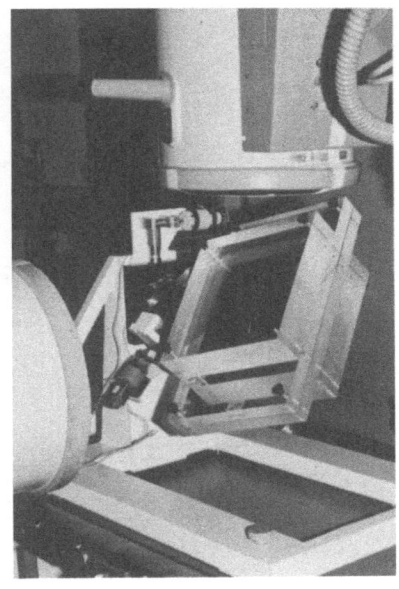

Fig. 2.4 Test-object for OTF-measurement.
Left: Frame with gold wires.   Right: Edge with scattering material.

The complex OTF_s is computed with its modulus (MTF_s) and phase (PTF_s)
as a function of spatial frequency. Strictly speaking, because the
system is not shift invariant, no OTF_s can be defined. In approximation,
however, an averaged OTF_s may be defined in patches with nearly constant
geometry. The location of these regions have been indicated in the insert of Fig. 2.6. The effect of stray radiation has been accounted for

---

[')] The design, based on suggestions by F. Timmer, has been effected
by I. van Egmond and the Mechanical Workshop of the Department of
Electrical Engineering: W. Bijleveld and G. Schotte.

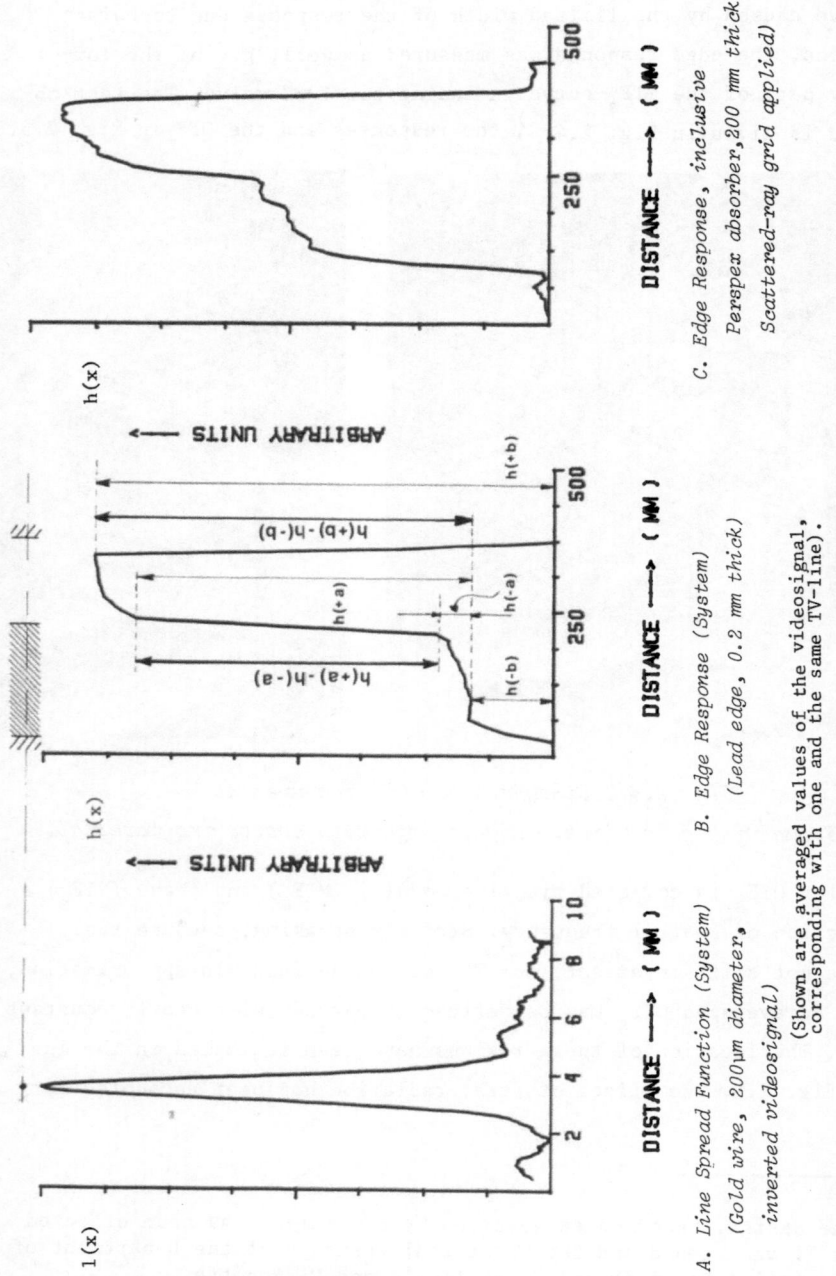

A. Line Spread Function (System)
   (Gold wire, 200µm diameter,
   inverted videosignal)

B. Edge Response (System)
   (Lead edge, 0.2 mm thick)
   (Shown are averaged values of the videosignal,
   corresponding with one and the same TV-line).

C. Edge Response, inclusive
   Perspex absorber,200 mm thick,
   Scattered-ray grid applied)

Fig. 2.5ᵃ Spatial Impulse and Edge Responses

26

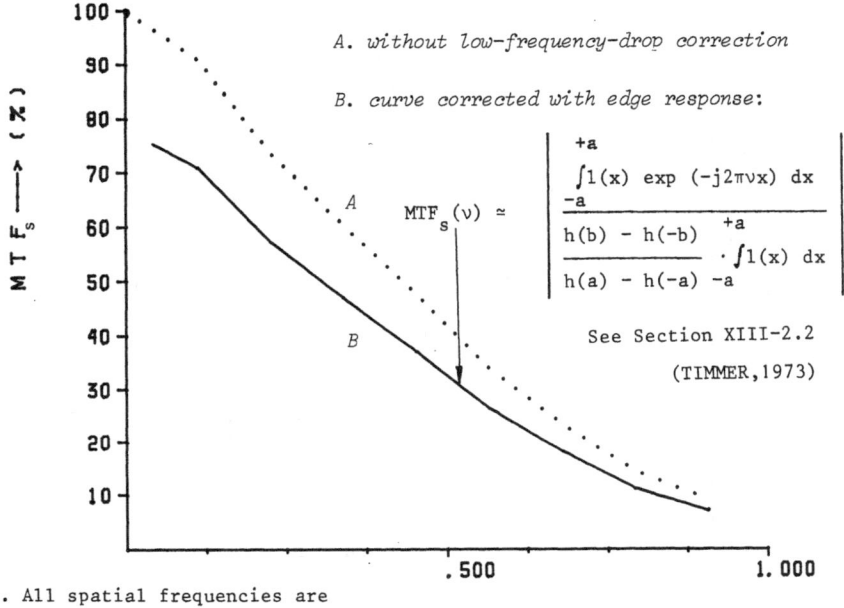

A. *without low-frequency-drop correction*

B. *curve corrected with edge response:*

$$MTF_s(\nu) \simeq \left| \frac{\int_{-a}^{+a} l(x) \exp(-j2\pi\nu x)\, dx}{\dfrac{h(b) - h(-b)}{h(a) - h(-a)} \cdot \int_{-a}^{+a} l(x)\, dx} \right|$$

See Section XIII-2.2

(TIMMER,1973)

N.B. All spatial frequencies are given with reference to the object plane.

Modulation Transfer Function

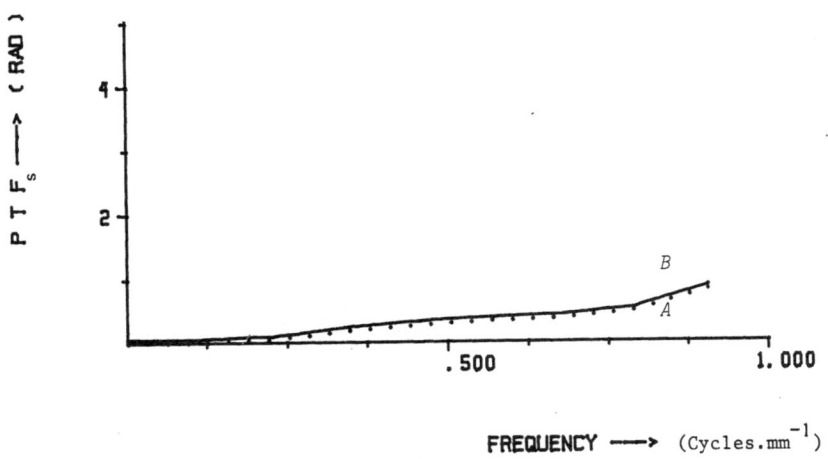

Phase Transfer Function

Fig. 2.5[b] Modulus and Phase of Optical Transfer Functions (X-ray tube - Image Intensifier - TV - System)

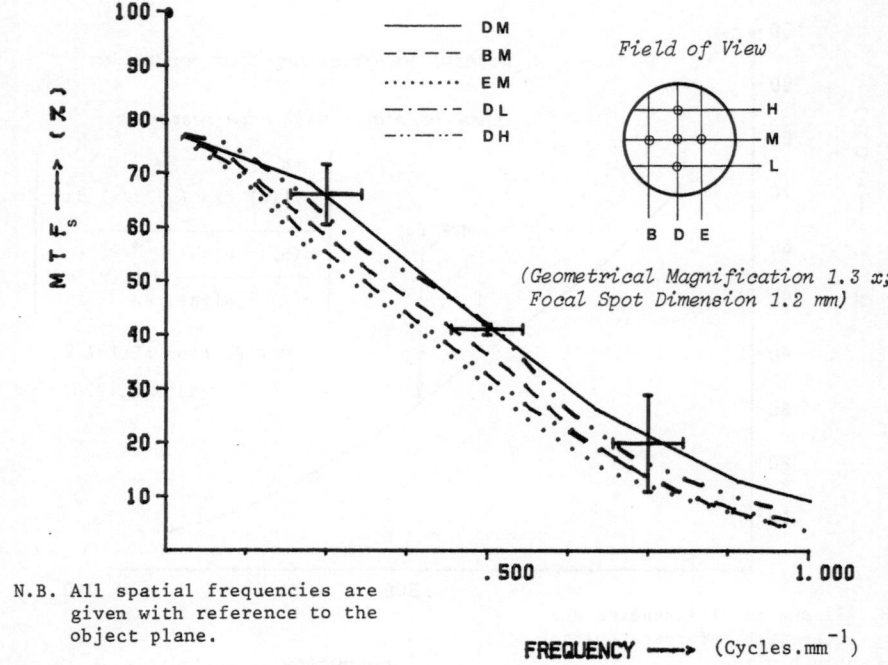

N.B. All spatial frequencies are
given with reference to the
object plane.

Modulation Transfer Functions

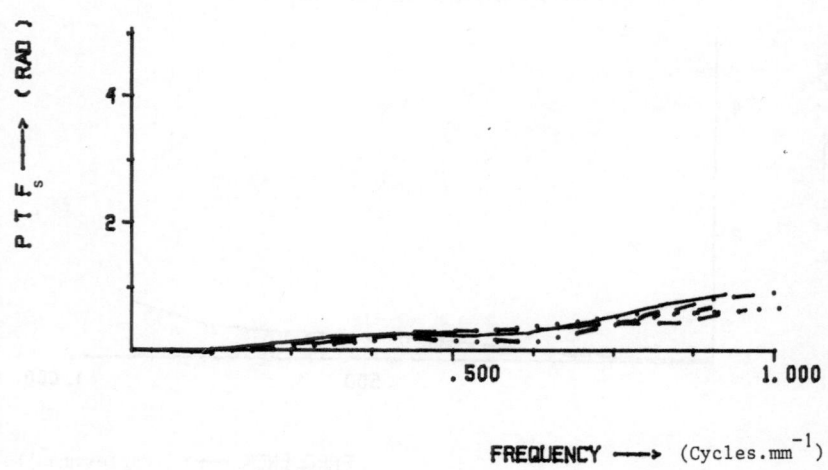

Phase Transfer Functions

Fig. 2.6ᵃ Deviation from Isoplanasy
(X-ray tube - Image Intensifier - TV - System)

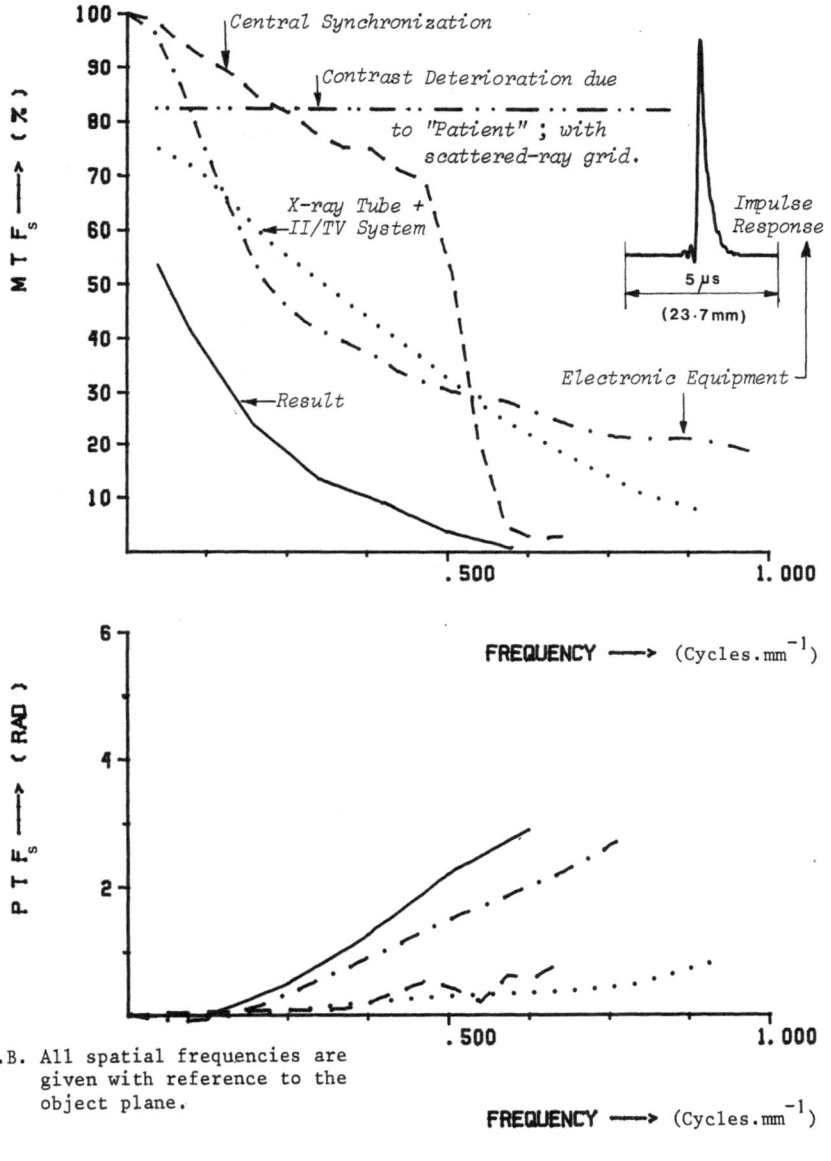

Fig. 2.6^b Influence of Additional Equipment

N.B. All spatial frequencies are
given with reference to the
object plane.

Thanks are due to F.Timmer and P.Bruin,Image Quality Group, Philips Medical
Systems Division, for their assistance in obtaining the curves of Figs. 2.5
and 2.6.

by a water-equivalent absorber of 20 cm thickness placed around the lead edge absorber. During this measurement, the BUCKY-filters have been inserted, to reproduce the situation as used in clinical practice. In this approach, the image deterioration caused by the system is judged on the basis of the amplitude spectrum of spatial frequencies describing the output image, compared with the input spectrum. The latter may be obtained by FOURIER analysis of microdensitographs (LISSNER,1968; SCOTT, 1969), or by calculations based on geometric models of the X-ray absorption (ROSSMAN,1969[a];1969[b]; ZISKIN,1971; KUNDEL,1972).

The temporal resolution has been measured with a rotating obturator as described by HERSTEL (1968). Two modulation depths have been realized by using absorbers as indicated in Fig. 2.7, together with the resulting MTF_t-curves. The output modulation has been measured by positioning a videodensitometer window at the relevant parts of the image.

In interpreting these curves with respect to our purpose, an estimate of the maximum posterior ventricular wall velocity component parallel to one of the imaging planes has to be used. LUDBROOK (1974) gives values of 37-56 mm.s^{-1} for patients with normal LV-function. We derived from echocardiograms[')] of four of such randomly chosen patients 49-80 mm.s^{-1}. As this velocity increases with heart rate, and dogs are used in our experiments, in formula (2.2) the relatively large value of $v = 100$ mm.s^{-1} has been used. From Fig. 6.3 a set of radii of curvature per slice as a function of the polar angle ψ has been derived, and minimum value of $R = 1,5$ mm chosen. Then, from the model according to ROSSMANN (1969[a]), as depicted in Fig. 13.1 a relevant spatial frequency spectrum $S(\nu)$ of the LV-shadow, can be estimated. So after the temporal frequency scale has been transformed into a spatial one, according to $\nu = f/v$, the image deterioration by temporal effects can be judged.

Besides by the characteristics of the system as mentioned above, the image is affected by the presence of noise. Analysis of the effects thereof would have been a study by itself. Several approaches have been

---

[')] Courteously put at our disposal by the Echocardiography Group, Thoraxcentre, Medical Faculty of the University of Rotterdam.

described (MOSELEY,1969). The resulting effect of the several types of noise present is implicly accounted for by the quantitative description of the human operator's overall performance to be given in section VII.3.

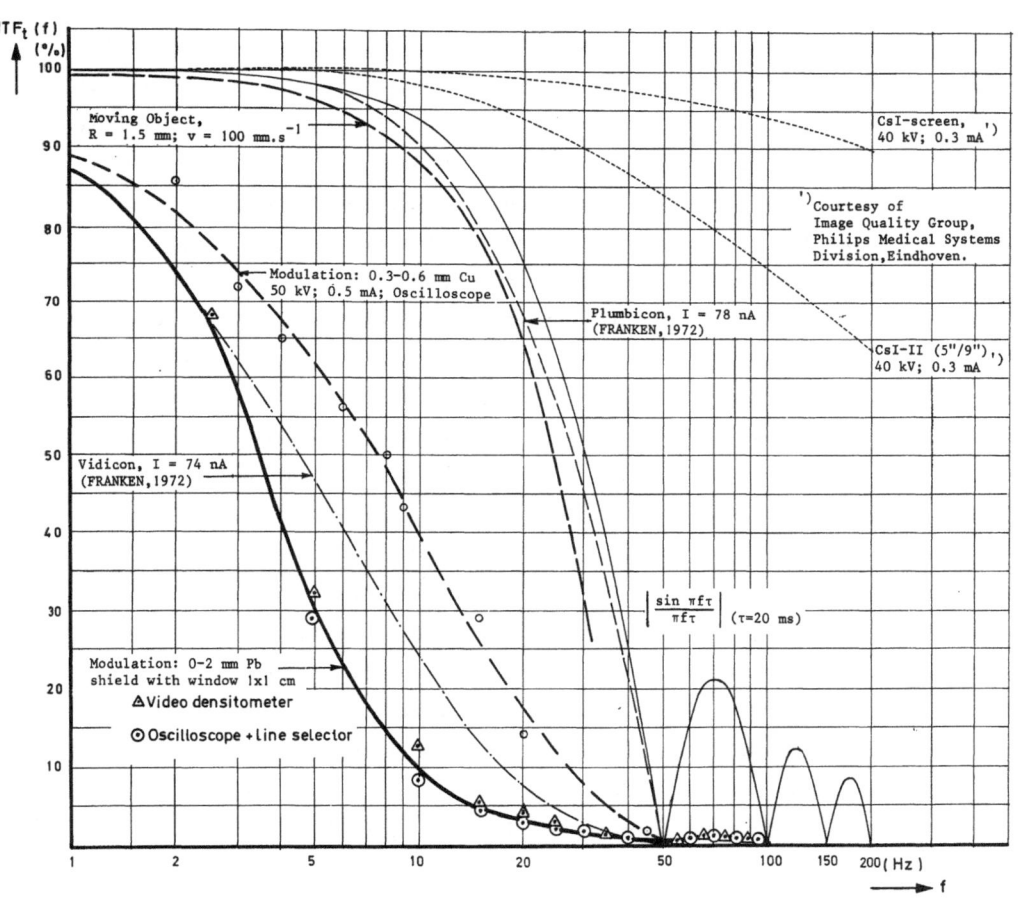

Fig. 2.7 Temporal Modulation Transfer Function Curves

[') Personal communication of G.Vijverberg and J.Proper.

31

4. Geometry in the Biplane Installation.

The left-ventricular cavity is a three-dimensional object, from which only the X-ray shadow projections can be obtained. In principle, a large number of projections are needed to give an adequate reconstruction. KIMURA (1973) uses X-ray pictures in six projections with 30° intervals by rotating the patient, taken at ES and ED moments as derived from the ECG. Subsequently, densitograms are taken along eleven lines perpendicular to the vertical axis of the cardiac shadow. Then, the total heart volume can be calculated by summation of the products of cross-sectional areas obtained by the cardiac silhouette as recognized by computer with the vertical distance of each division. JOHNSON (1973) *et.al.* claim to be able to obtain quite accurate three-dimensional reconstructions of irregularly shaped nonhomogeneous structures, such as the intact heart, by a large number of multiplane X-ray projections, which are submitted to high-resolution videodensitometry. Both procedures must impose a considerable dose burden to the patient, and may therefore not be applicable routinely. Methods in use for three-dimensional object reconstruction from a limited number of projections are: FOURIER synthesis (CROWTHER, 1970[a],1970[b]), holography (REDMAN,1968), Monte Carlo- and algebraic methods (FRIEDER,1971; GORDON,1971). Because of instrumentation and patient dose limitations, only orthogonal biplane projections are used in clinical practice. Since, in principle, it is not possible to reconstruct an arbitrary three-dimensional object from two projections, certain assumptions must be made on the shape (CHANG,1971[a],1971[b],1973); which will be discussed in more detail in Chapter VI.

A second reason why at least a biplane installation is required in quantitative angiocardiography, is, that the position of the heart inside the body has to be measured in order to be able to calculate the magnification factors of the divergent projections. Simultaneous exposure in sagittal and frontal directions for this purpose came into use in 1932-1935 (LYSHOLM,1934; JONSELL,1939). The divergent X-ray beams produce a shadow pattern on the sensitive screens of the image intensifiers with projective enlargement. The corresponding magnification factors can be

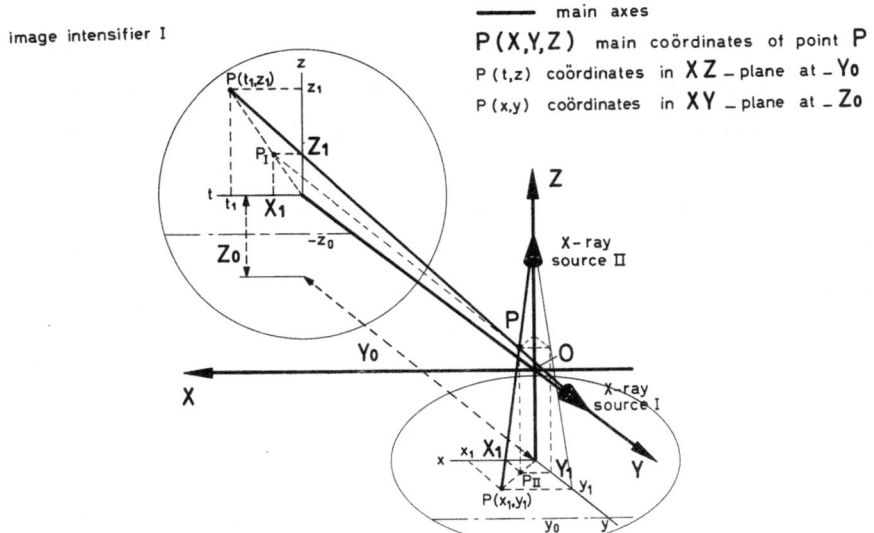

image intensifier I

main axes

$P(X,Y,Z)$ main coördinates of point P

$P(t,z)$ coördinates in XZ _ plane at _ Y_0

$P(x,y)$ coördinates in XY _ plane at _ Z_0

image intensifier II

A. THREE DIMENSIONAL

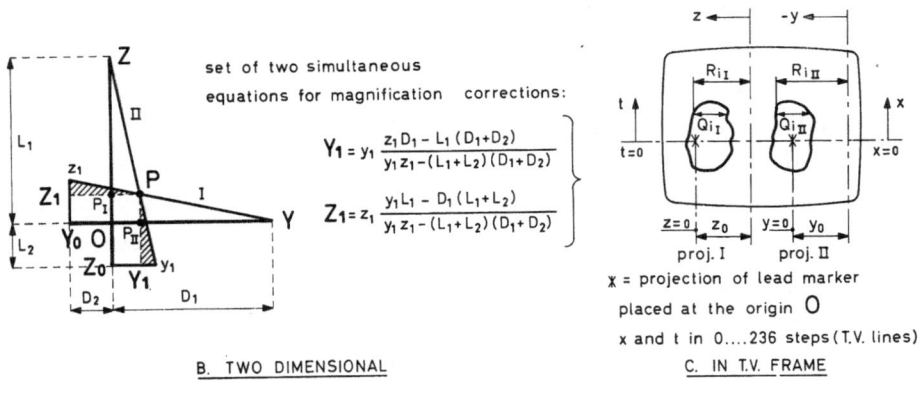

set of two simultaneous

equations for magnification corrections:

$$Y_1 = y_1 \frac{z_1 D_1 - L_1 (D_1 + D_2)}{y_1 z_1 - (L_1 + L_2)(D_1 + D_2)}$$

$$Z_1 = z_1 \frac{y_1 L_1 - D_1 (L_1 + L_2)}{y_1 z_1 - (L_1 + L_2)(D_1 + D_2)}$$

$\mathbf{x}$ = projection of lead marker

placed at the origin O

x and t in $0....236$ steps (T.V. lines)

B. TWO DIMENSIONAL

C. IN T.V. FRAME

BIPLANE PROJECTIONS

Fig. 2.8 (After NELSON, 1966).

calculated if the position of the heart relative to the main axes is
known. As shown in Fig. 2.8., based on NELSON (1966), the coordinates
(X,Y) of a point P in orthogonal projection can be derived from its
measured projection coordinates (y,z) with magnification factors which
are functions of both y and z and the known distances D_1,L_1 resp. D_2,L_2
of the X-ray tube foci and image intensifier input screens respective
to the main axes. So a set of two simultaneous equations has to be solved
for each point to calculate the true dimensions of the left ventricle
from the shadow projections (STEWART,1968; BOVE,1970[a]). The quantities
D_1,D_2,L_1 and L_2 are measured with steel bands, attached to the telescop-
ic supports of the X-ray tubes and image intensifiers.

A problem is, that the formulae given apply only to pairs of measured
points of which it is known that these are the projections of one and
the same point in space. This generally does not hold true for biplane
contour point pairs. DODGE (1960) used the method to calculate both the
spatial direction and magnitude of a defined line (ventricle long axis)
from the two X-ray projections. After two minor axes in an ellipsoidal
model for the LV have been computed from the areas enclosed by the contours in both projections, the true end-points of these axes can be reconstructed according to the same principle by a computer program developed
by NELSON (1966). It had already been shown by ARVIDSSON (1957), that
even with a geometrically defined ellipsoid the volume cannot be determined with the aid of two orthogonal projections if the orientation of
the axes is not known. The long axis of the LV has been determined by
the same author (1961) from these projections; with a constant magnification factor, however. GOERKE (1967) uses an enlargement factor corresponding with the calculated center of mass of the cardiac cavity, whereas the image of the catheter tip within the left ventricle is exploited
for this purpose by MARCUS (1972). As will be shown in Chapter IX,
section 3, we use a different magnification factor for each section of
the LV-cavity, based on the corresponding division point of the long
axis in true spatial position.

5. Calibration.

The calculations, mentioned in the preceding section, assume:

a. Perpendicular intersection of the main axes of the X-ray image intensifier system, and

b. Projection on entrance windows of the image intensifiers which are planes perpendicular to these main axes.

Although there is a vast amount of literature on LVV-determination by biplane angiocardiography, we found only two publications mentioning their adjustment procedure which is essential to the method. SCHOHL (1971) and HEINTZEN (1971[c]) use a combination of a plummet with two lead spheres and a water-levelling instrument from a U-tube filled with contrast medium, as marking arrows on the frames proved unreliable for a proper adjustment. A plastic cube with 7 cm edge on which small metal discs have been glued is used to give both X-ray systems equal magnification. According to SCHOHL, in this approach the ventricle under investigation should be placed within a region of $\pm$ 5 cm from the intersection point of the beams. This seems less useful, as it limits the clinician in the positioning of the patient. A phantom, consisting of an alumina frame with lead beads on steel wires along the side and body diagonals is used by STEWART (1968). Our solution for the problem *sub a* is the X-ray aiming device as depicted in Fig. 2.9[a], consisting of a hollow plastic cube of 25 cm edge, on the accurately machined planes of which specially formed lead markers have been glued. Fig. 2.9[b] shows the X-ray shadows in both projections on the TV-screen. A misadjustment of 2 mm is still discernible on the monitor screen, and corresponds with an angular error of about 5 minutes in an average situation.

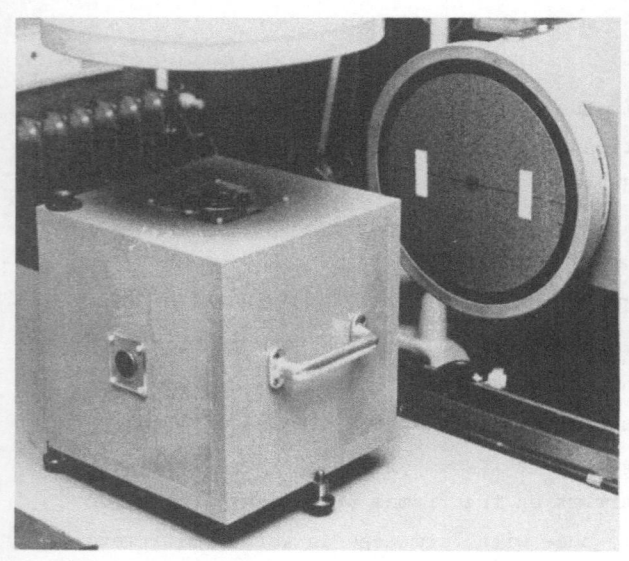
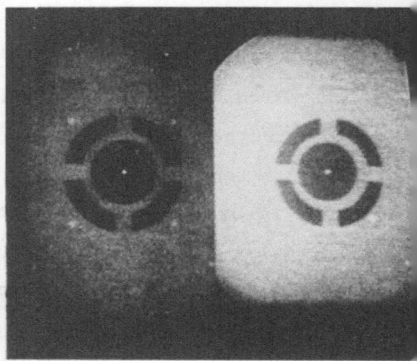

Fig. 2.9

X-ray Aiming Device
Left: The device positioned, note the waterlevelling instrument.
Right: The corresponding TV-picture.

Several methods have been described to account for the fact that the
entrance window of an image intensifier is spherical rather than flat,
causing the assumption mentioned *sub b* are to be incorrect. STEWART
(1968) checked the spatial linearity of the imaging system with a steel
disc, placed at the entrance window of the image intensifier under
study. A pattern of holes along radii spaced $22\frac{1}{2}^{\circ}$ with a distance of
1 cm proved to reproduce with errors of 12 to 13% at radii of 5 to 6 cm
and growing with the radius. The circular symmetry was retained, however,
as might be expected from the cylindrical construction of image intensifiers. A third order correction polynome was used to correct this distortion. The method had been first described by BARRY (1963). Another
approach has been used by KASSER (1969), who superimposed to the picture
a 1x1 cm^2 cross-hatched grid, filmed at the same position relative to

the image intensifier as the ventricle studied. The number of squares superimposed on the LV-shadow was counted, and the total area plani-metered. The square root of the ratio of both areas then could be used for correcting both X-ray magnification and distortion.

A method to determine absolute dimensions in X-ray projections by parallax after a known displacement of the patient in a direction per-pendicular to the projection axis (telediametry) has been described by BUECHNER (1968). The device, consisting of a set of servocontrolled cas-settes containing reference marks and a continuously stretchable ruler with radiopaque inscriptions, is commercially available. A drawback is that adjustment has to be done under X-ray illumination. Calibration of the data conversion part of our system was achieved with metal masks, placed on the image intensifier entrance windows. In these masks, cir-cular slits are cut with different radii and .25 mm width. If X-ray beams are applied, the resulting videosignal is of sufficiently high contrast to be directly accepted by the video-computer interface. Thus the number of counts in the computer input corresponding with the sampled points are known. After calculation of the mean square best-fit of the circle through these points, the calibration in horizontal

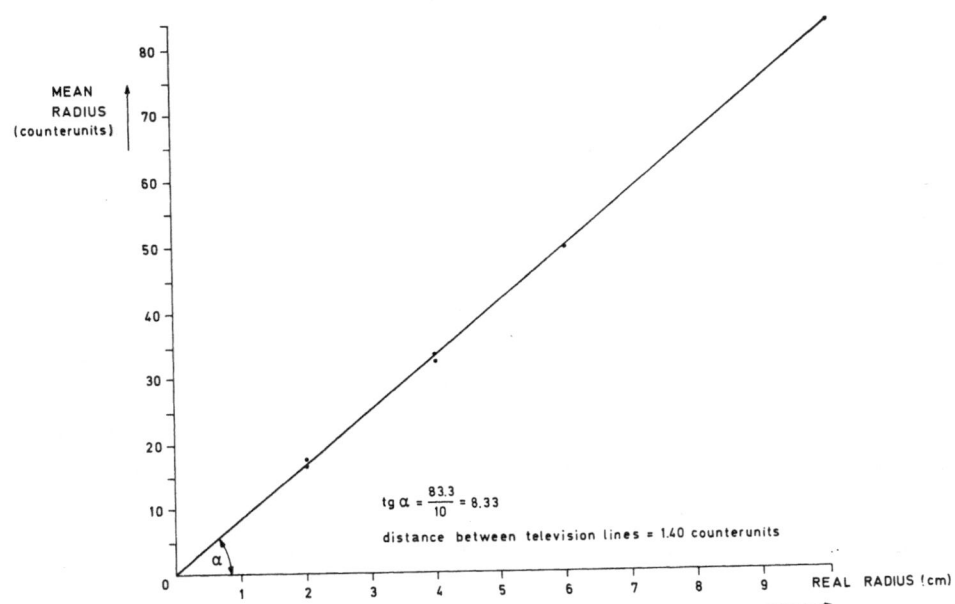

Fig. 2.10 Calibration Curve

37

(number of counts per mm) and in vertical direction (number of counts per distance between successive TV-lines) is established. The results are shown in Fig. 2.10.

In our system, two test frames are taken at the end of each measurement with the position of the X-ray tubes and image intensifiers unchanged. The first contains pictures of one of the circular slit masks described before. The centres of the circles found from the least-squares best fit are considered to be the projections of the origin of the main coordinate system. The second one contains the shadow of a metal sphere of accurately known volume; the contours of this test object has to be drawn by the human observer. This calibration of the measurement system in terms of volume is chosen because besides the easy availability of accurately machined balls, one of the geometric models frequently use for LVV calculation (see Chapter VI) is exact for a spheroid. SCHOHL (1972) and CHAPMAN (1958) thus found a relative difference in the order of -0,5% with respect to the known volume. A survey on the statistical results from a study of the accuracy of the different steps in a biplane videometric measurement system using various test models has been published by HEINTZEN (1971[d]), partly based on the work of VOGEL (1971). A test sphere with a volume about equal to that of the ventricle measured, to be positioned such that its shadow appears at the same region as the ventricular projections, has been used by ZIMMERMAN (1973) to eliminate the influence of unequal projection factors. The use of such a general correction factor in a biplane system, while a digital computer is used for LVV calculation, seems oversimplistic with regard to the sophistication of the installation.

At the end of this chapter, it is stressed once more, that the silhouttes on the image intensifier input screens are obtained by *central shadow projection*. This means that the X-ray beams tangent to a structure determine the contour thereof, so small raised rims have a relatively large influence on the contour, and concave regions are not shown. For this reason, the matematical model used in reconstructing the volume and shape of the depicted organ should account for these effects by a fairly detailed description of the general shape of the organ. In Chapter VI such a model will be proposed for the left ventricular cavity.

III. FRACTIONIZED CONTRAST MEDIUM INJECTION

1. *Introduction*

Selective angiocardiography of the left ventricle makes use of the injection of a radiopaque medium into the ventricle itself or at a point
upstream into the central circulation. TIMM (1947) was the first to
opacify the left ventricle and to record the ventricular movement as
well as its mixing characteristics by means of roentgencinematography.
The technique of catheterization of the heart cavities has been developed to a sophisticated level (PORSTMANN,1962). The injection of contrast medium through catheters has been investigated by OLIN (1963), the
intermittent injection technique is described in detail by SCHAD (1967).
Several types of electromechanical injectors have become commercially
available since. Investigation of the flow characteristics of injection
catheters (KROVETZ,1966; BOVE,1968; SUSMAN,1969) has led to the development of flow-controlled injectors.

One of the main problems in quantitative angiocardiography is the
modification of the circulation caused by the contrast medium injected.
The sudden addition of volume to the left ventricle increases the ventricular size (HALLERMAN,1964). To prevent this, the total allowable
amount of contrast medium to be administered has to be injected in a

number of portions as small as is consistent with the detectability of
the contour of the LV shadow. All contrast agents generate myocardial
hypoxia as an amount of blood is displaced by a solution which contains
no oxygen (DEAN,1966). A second important cause of influence on the
heart function is a change in osmolality (ISERI,1965; KLOSTER,1967).
Adverse reactions to contrast agents have been reported in general
(ANSELL,1970) and with respect to haemodynamic responses (LINDGREN,1970;
GOOTMAN,1970), especially myocardial contractility (BLINKS,1963). In
connection with left ventricular volume measurements, it is concluded
by CARLETON (1971) that:

> *"Efforts to measure left ventricular performance using angiocardio-*
> *graphy may be focused on the first 2 and possibly 3 cardiac cycles*
> *after the beginning of left ventricular opacification. Data derived*
> *from cardiac cycles after this point in time may no longer reflect*
> *the previously existing state of cardiac performance."*

Thus, the administration of the fractions of contrast medium has to be
programmed, as the changes last for several minutes. A comparison of the
LVV as determined by angiography with the volume obtained from the position of six endocardial lead beads (MITCHELL,1967) by means of an ellipsoid model according to MULLINS (1972), has led to the same conclusion.
After the volume load-effect caused by the injection itself, firstly a
deterioration of LV-function (fall in max. dP/dt) occurred, and secondly
a transient increase which lasted about 15 minutes.

Basing himself on a literature survey, BARON (1973) criticizes the
angiographic method of ejection fraction (EF) determination for not resulting in a significantly smaller borderline group of patients to be
selected for coronary arterial surgery, compared with the group in which
the conclusions are based on experienced observation of the cineangio-
cardiogram. Moreover the frequent occurrence of extra-systoles induced
mechanically by the force of the fluid jets during contrast injection
(KROVETZ,1970) induce alterations in myocardial function also.
So, measurement techniques based on angiocardiography tend to violate the
principle that the subject under investigation should not be altered by
the measurement procedure. Moreover, the total allowable amount of contrast medium as related to body weight, mostly 3 mg per kg, is another

limiting factor in the investigation. In section 4 of this chapter a procedure will be described to administer this quantity in portions at predetermined moments in the cardiac cycle in such a way that a maximum number of videoframes containing the LV-shadow in sufficient contrast can be obtained. This implies that the catheter, injection pressure and flow have to be chosen in order to diminish the probability of extra-systoles caused by direct mechanical stimulation.

2. *Calculation of the Number of Fractions*

The contrast medium used in the clinic, "Isopaque Coronar® 75%" [1], is a sodium salt of metrizoate which has been introduced in 1966 by DAHLSTROEM, and features a low viscosity with the absence of contra-indication in digitalized patients (SALVESEN,1966). Details of the medium have been published by the importer (PHARMACHEMIE,1968); its structure formula reads:

The atomic composition has been measured [2] to be in relative weight:

Element	Z	Rel.weight
Hydrogen	1	0.0690
Carbon	6	0.1495
Nitrogen	7	0.0317
Oxygen	8	0.4829
Iodine	53	0.2669

Table 3.1

The density at 37 degrees centigrade is $\rho = 1.393$ g.cm^{-3}; the X-ray contrast is mostly due to the iodine content, as shown in table 3.2 in section XIII-4. The viscosity amounts to 6.6 cP at the same temperature if the solution acts as a NEWTONIAN fluid. The good solubility in water of 86g per 100 ml is assured because of the fact that it is a sodium salt of the relevant acid.

---

[1] Manufacturer: Nyegaard, Oslo; Importer, Pharmachemie, Haarlem
[2] Physisch Chemisch Instituut TNO

The degree of opacity brought about by a contrast medium in an organ of given dimensions depends on the linear extinction coefficient μ (cm^{-1}) and its density ρ ($g.cm^{-3}$). Exept for a sudden increase at the absorption edges, μ decreases rapidly with the photon energy E of the radiation. For iodine, with a K-absorption limit at 33.2 keV, a maximum in μ is found at 34 keV radiation, even larger than that of much heavier elements (OOSTERKAMP,1961[a]). STRID (1973) has shown, that for a composite substance of density ρ, $\mu(E)$ is proportional to ρ, for all photon energies E in the range used for radiography. If the contrast medium is composed of n weight fractions a_i of elements with mass absorption coefficients $(\frac{\mu}{\rho})_{Z_i}$, the total mass absorption coefficient μ/ρ is found to be, according to MELLINK (1961):

$$\frac{\mu}{\rho} = \sum_{i=1}^{n} a_i \left(\frac{\mu}{\rho}\right)_{Z_i} \quad , \text{ with } \sum_{i=1}^{n} a_i = 1 \quad \ldots \ldots \ldots \ldots \ldots (3.2)$$

To make use of these relationships in the case of polychromatic radiation the energy spectrum $I_o(E)$ has to be taken into account, and an effective linear extinction coefficient $\bar{\mu}$ may be calculated according to SCHOKNECHT (1966):

$$e^{-\bar{\mu}D} \int_0^{\infty} I_o(E)dE = \int_0^{\infty} I_o(E)e^{-\mu(E)D} dE \ldots \ldots \ldots \ldots \ldots (3.3)$$

in which D is the thickness of a homogeneous layer, irradiated perpendicularly. A mathematical model of contrast formation including the emission of the tube target, the absorption process, and the conversion of the absorption relief into an image has been published by STRID (1973), the computed data have been compared with experimentally measured values by LANTZ (1973). Characterization of radiation quality by one "effective wavelength" has been discussed by WOLSCHENDORF (1973) for low-energy radiation. The underlying theoretical considerations have been discussed by HEINTZEN in general (1971[h]) and with the use of pulsed radiation (1971[i]). In the latter case, it is concluded that for a range of tube voltages between 50 and 90 kV and within other limits the validity regions of LAMBERT-BEER's law in roentgendensitometry of contrast medium using pulsed radiation as described by BUERSCH (1972) still hold (MOLDENHAUER,1972), in his experimental situation.

In the considerations mentioned above, the aspect of contrast detectability has not yet been taken into account. By LYSELL (1968), the gamma of photographic film has been considered in low-contrast cases. Aspects of the perception of details in X-ray pictures came into discussion by SCHOBER (1966) in general, and by ROEHLER (1969) with respect to noise, presentation time, and repetition frequency. Contrast sensitivity functions are discussed as aids in the description of vision by VAN MEETEREN (1973). A contrast difference of 2 to 4% in the regions to be discerned is given as a rule-of-thumb by MELLINK (1961).

The contrast on the image intensifier input screen is smaller than that in the primary radiation due to scattering in the thorax (SEEMAN, 1968). The same author gives a survey of factors affecting radiographic detail, as does FEDDEMA (1969). The usefulness of grids to reduce scattered X-rays may be expressed in a quality factor (HONDIUS BOLDINGH, 1964). In many cases, the small number of different grids available and the additional radiation dose required limit a specific application. The percentage of scattered radiation exposure rate in the outgoing beam has not been found described in detail; from STIEVE (1966[b]) and SPIEGLER (1957), a rough taxation of 80% has been chosen by SNEEK in his calculation of the maximum number of fractions in which this medium can be administered in the case of an estimated relative volume error of 1%. The model used and the assumptions made are described in detail in section XIII-2. In the case of a sphere, the difference in volume has been calculated from the known and detected diameters, the latter depend on the contrast at the border. This contrast is determined by the concentration of contrast medium and the energy spectrum of the radiation, corresponding with a chosen tube voltage.

The results are depicted in Fig. 3.1, which gives the volume concentration of contrast medium as a function of the tube voltage with the diameter of the spherical model as a parameter (SNEEK,internal report M82). From these curves, the concentration to be used in practice may be derived with the help of measurements on LV-cast sections, as shown in Fig. 8.3. From the minimal radius or curvature together with the tube voltage the concentration to be used can be chosen. In general, this concentration is of the order of 8%, meaning that the total permissible amount of contrast medium as based on body weight, can be injected in 8 fractions. (Dog, 10 kg; EDV = 50 ml; 3 ml contrast medium per kg).

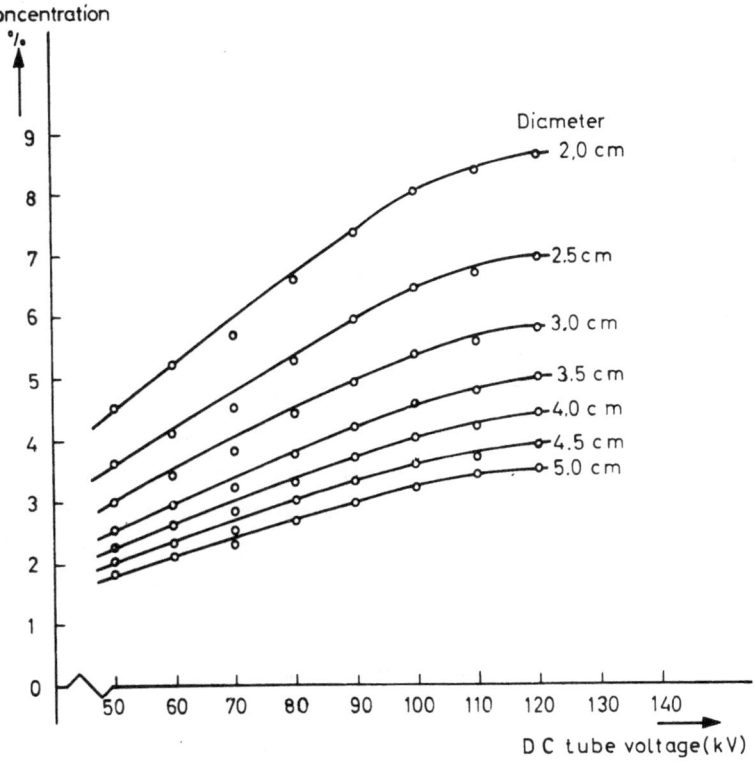

Fig. 3.1 *Concentration vs Tube Voltage Curves* *(SNEEK,1971).*

3. Experimental Determination of the Concentration of Medium

In the preceding section, simplifying assumptions have been made with
regard to the homegeneity of the contrast medium. The actual situation
is more intricate because of the viscosity of the medium, which precludes instant mixing. Injection into the ventricle during early diastole is used to obtain the best possible circumstances; intermittent
injection may be performed to obtain an opacity level as desired during
some heartbeats (SCHAD,1967). The effects on cardiac function as mentioned in section III-1, *e.g.* by KROVETZ (1970) contraindicate a pro-
longed injection period. Also a smooth endocardial wall has been assumed
in the sphere model, whereas there are many small cavities between the
trabeculae carneae in which the blood-contrast medium mixture will not
deliver a sufficiently high contrast.

Marking of the LV-cavity outline does not necessarily have to be performed with a liquid. If the exact position of isolated points on the
epicardial or endocardial wall suffices, small metal markers may be used
in the experimental animal or even in patients which have undergone
thoracic surgery (HARRISON,1963; MACDONALD,1970). Also lead coating of
the tricuspid valve in dogs has been described (CARLSSON,1964). Marker
pairs connected with an elastic string have been used for measuring
regional myocardial movement as well as wall thickness (HEIKKILA,1972).
Six lead beads, sutured on the endocardial wall at proper places are
used to demarcate the end-points of the major and the two minor axes
of an assumed ellipsoidal shell of cardiac muscle adjacent to the cavity
of the left ventricle in dogs by MITCHELL (1967); WILDENTHAL (1969); and
LESHIN (1972). After the operation, measurements may be performed on the
animal in an unanaesthetized state to determine left ventricular ellipsoidal cavity volume and area as well as axial lenghts, circumferences,
and wall thickness (with the use of additional epicardial clips;
MITCHELL,1969). A technique in which open-chest surgery is obviated has
been described by CARLSSON (1967). Tantalum wire spirals of 2 mm long
and 0.12 mm wide are introduced through a bending-tip catheter and

screwed into the endocardial wall with a flexible "screw-driver" wire.
Besides a demonstration of the extension of the cloud of contrast medium
injected in angiocardiography and changes in LV-function produced thereby (MULLINS,1972), the marked dogs were also used to determine motion
curves of the relevant points in the myocardial wall (CARLSSON,1969;
1970), as well as diastolic pressure-volume relationships, plastic, vis-
cous and inertial properties of the left ventricle in diastole (NOBLE,
1969[a]). The tantalum screw markers have also been used to check the method suggested by KONG (1971) in which the position of coronary artery
bifurcations is determined with angiography (DAUGHTERS,1973), to measure
instantaneous epicardial segmental length. This has also been investigated by optical methods using glass fibers. INGELS (1971) concluded
from such measurements that regional myocardial dynamic behaviour is not
dictated solely by regional fiber orientation, but that the ventricular
fibers must be viewed as functional bundles as well.

During experiments using extracorporal circulation in dogs in the
Laboratory for Experimental Cardiology at Utrecht, left-ventricular
marking during open-chest surgery has been used.
This procedure was chosen as the introduction of the CARLSSON technique
in this laboratory required costly modification of the steering catheters
in use. Special markers and applicators as shown in Fig. 3.2 were used[').
The markers consist of silvered cylinders of a bismuth alloy["), with
stainless steel springs, the depth of application is fixed by the impact
disks at the end of the *cannulae* during extraxtion of the applicator,

[')Thanks are due to N.J Minekus and J. van der Sluis of the workshop
for precision mechanical techniques of the University of Technology
for the development of these devices

["]Brand: Cerromatrix; Manufacturer: Mining & Chemical Prducts
(London)

the markers are kept in place by means of a steel wire mounted on the piston. After recovery of the dog, X-ray pictures were taken with various concentrations of contrast medium. Our purpose has been to establish the accuracy of LV-cavity outline determination from the contrast "cloud" injected. As the markers had "travelled" into the myocard, their position relative to the endocardial wall had to be determined by separate X-ray pictures of the excised heart as shown in Fig. 3.3. The results confirmed those of section III-2, measurements on cylindrical phantoms described by Sneek (internal report M82), reproduced in Table 3.3 (section XIII-4), supported this evidence.

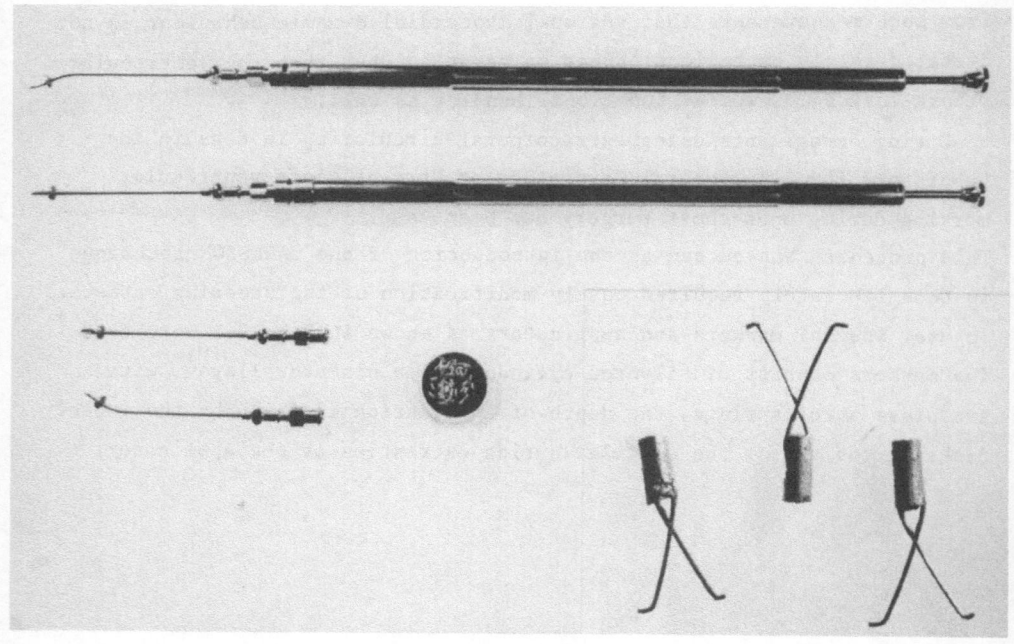

Fig. 3.2 *Markers and Applicators*
Straight as well as bended cannulae are used
for the application of markers. Total length
of applicators is about 30 cm.
Insert: markers in detail.
Length of cylinders is about 2 mm.

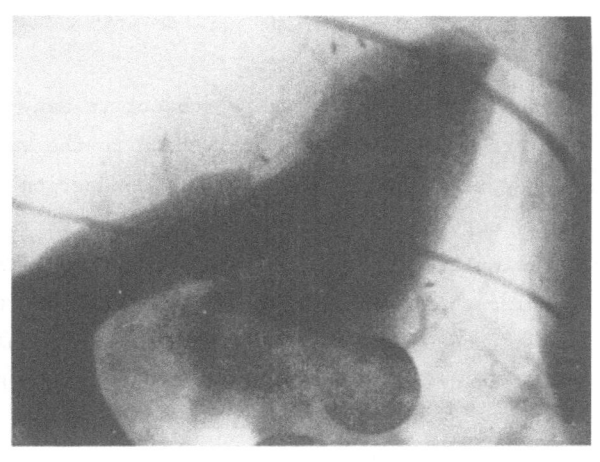

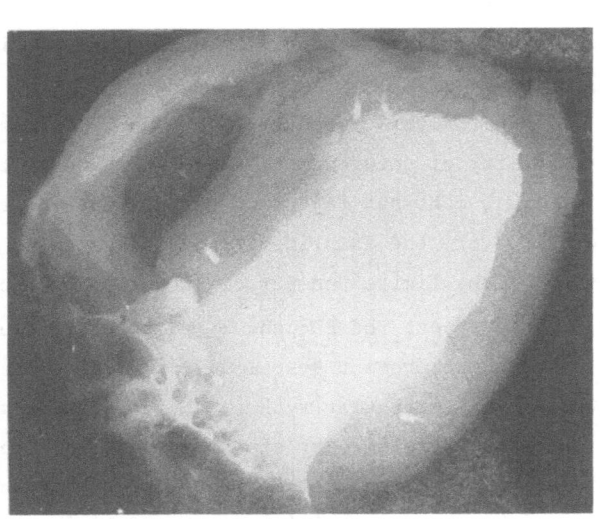

Fig. 3.3 *Extension of Contrast Cloud Relative to Markers*
Left: X-ray picture of excised heart with markers.
Right: Single picture of cineangiogram in corresponding
view, showing the extension of the contrast medium.

4. Time Programming

In the normal heart, activation of the auricles is subject to many
physiologic variables. The transmission of the activation to the ventricles includes a time delay regulated by the specific conduction system (HEETHAAR,1972). This is especially a problem in the case atrial
fibrillation is present or simulated by a stimulation programme. Atrial
fibrillation gives rise to irregular ventricular contractions, due to
effects of atrial impulses on conduction through the atrio-ventricular
node. This phenomenon can be described by a statistical model (TEN HOOPEN,
1966), and explained by scaling of the rate of atrial impulses by the
atrio-ventricular conduction system (BOOTSMA,1970). In the experimental
situation, findings during artificial atrial fibrillation cannot be used
without reserve to explain electrophysiological or haemodynamic phenomena
in true artial fibrillation (STRACKEE,1971). The effect of sudden changes
in heart rate on LVV in dogs has been measured by thermodilution with
a fast-response bead thermistor by BRISTOW (1963). NOBLE (1969[b]) investigated the effect of heart rate on myocardial contractility as represented by the maximal time derivative of the LV-pressure, and concluded
that the interval-strength relationship has a plateau at the physiological range of heart rate. End diastolic segment length, the interval-
strength relationship and aortic systolic pressure (preload, contrac-
tillity, and afterload) may be studied effectively during atrial fibrillation (KARLINER,1974).

Angiocardiographic methods for this purpose present difficulties.
Because of the unpredictability of occurence of the R-wave and of the
duration of the next interval, contrast injection during diasole at fixed
intervals is precluded. Moreover, the sampling of the images takes place
with a fixed frequency so of the limited number of pictures to be taken
only a small fraction will represent the ED- and ES-moments to be used
for calculation of SV. As the measurement system described here has been
built to be used in studies with irregular rythms, an intricate time-
programming system is essential. Preliminary experiments using fluoroscopy
and photocameras with electrical shutter, also with photographic subtraction have been performed with a hardware timing system of limited faciliti

When the use of video methods and pulsed X-rays became pertinent, a more flexible timing unit proved necessary. A hardware simulator, implemented on a reprogrammable microcomputer [), has been designed and interfaced to the various apparatus as shown in Fig. 3.4. This device is compatible with a conventional teletype for programming and providing hard copy records. The output is decoded and fed to the control devices of the videodisk, stimulator, contrast injector, and X-ray pulsing equipment. The timing of the ES- and ED-moments is governed by electric pulses supplied to the time programming unit. For the ED-moment, an analog R-wave detector is used, which contains a triggering circuit preceded by a band-pass filter and an automatic voltage control circuit. The ES-moment is found from the first time derivative of the LV-pressure curve; a more accurate timing is obtained from simultaneously measured left ventricular and aortic pressure curves, together with a time window positioned by the R-wave (internal report M91). If only the SV = EDV-ESV is required, the relevant videoframe can be automatically selected from markings on the second audiochannel of a videotaperecorder, and copied on the videodisk semi-automatically (internal report M104).

As videosubtraction is used in our system, pictures reflecting the heart in the same state of contraction, but with and without added contrasts have to be recorded on different channels but at the same track number of the videodisk as described in section IV-3. The facility for this procedure is also comprised in the timing system, but requires artificial stimulation of the heart. With the help of a special iterative programme, the time intervals between the stimuli, which produce the RR-intervals required, have to be determined. Next, a sequence of the latter has to be established in order to obtain as much information as possible from the limited number of injections.

[) INTEL MCS4/SIM 4-01. *Suggested and programmed by J.H.J. Sneek.*

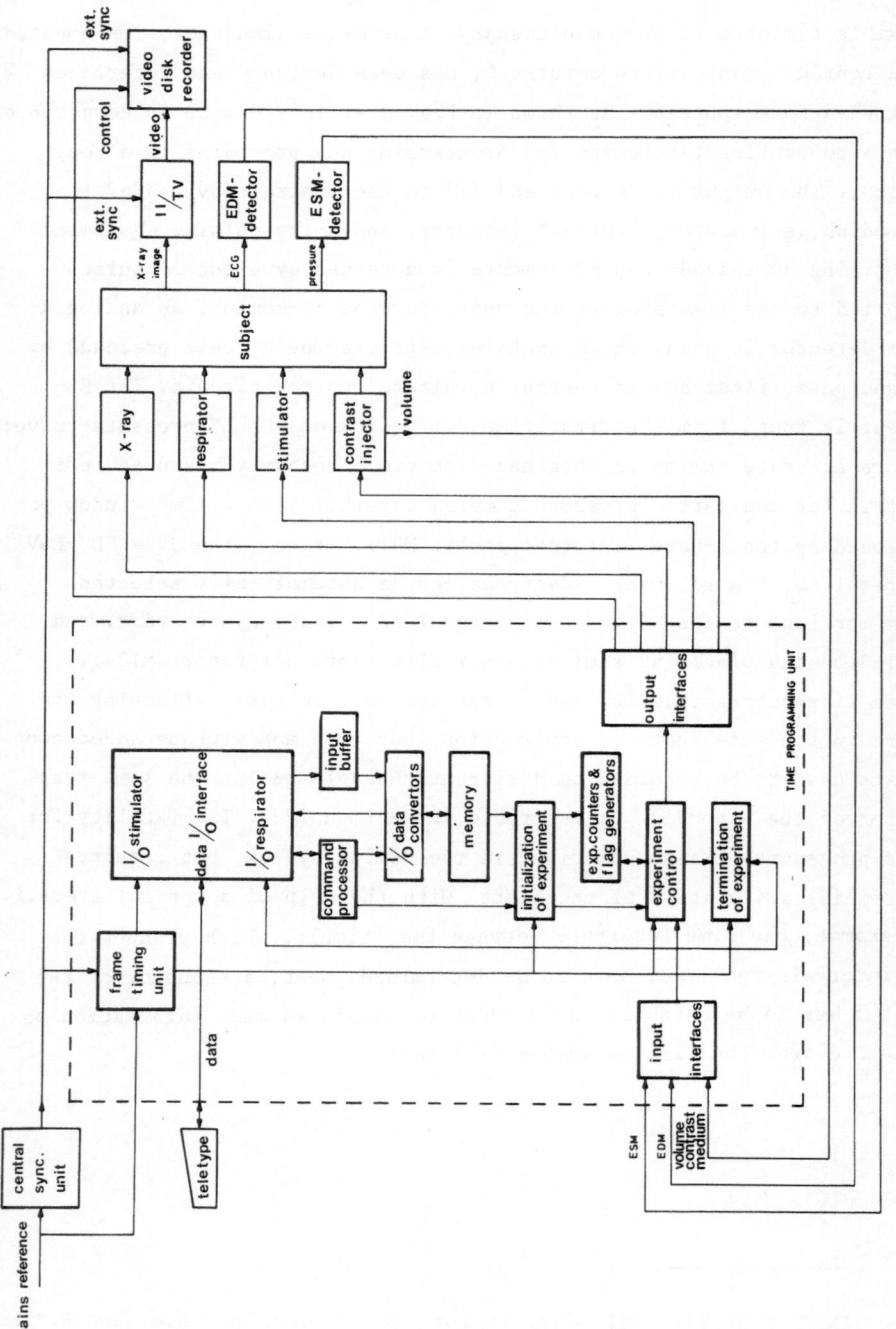

Fig. 3.4 Time Programming System

5. *Radiation Dose*

Because of the irreversibility of biological changes provoked by X-rays, the radiation dose administered to the patient has to be considered in relation to the information gained by the radiological method used for diagnosis. The ratio of the image quality (defined in terms of spatial resolution), SCHOTT (1961), or information index (the product of contrast sensitivity and resolution), FRIEDELL (1965), to the patient dose have been suggested as measures for the effectiveness of radiological procedures. The attempt of our investigation is to increase the diagnostic information gained by the cardiac catheterization procedure without increasing the dose as given to the patient during conventional diagnostic procedures. This is effected by controlling the formation as well as the evaluation of the videoangiocardiograms. A dose reduction is to be expected, even if the dose per radiation pulse is not smaller than the dose administered during one frame by continuous irradiation, by using a videodisk, thus separating exposure and interpretation (BAKER, 1967). The image may be obtained by radiation pulses of about 2 ms duration, while the averaging time of the eye is about 200 ms, depending on the screen luminance. Besides, the observer has only a limited region of sharp focus (FRIEDELL, 1965).

Radiation dose to patients undergoing cardiac catherization has always been considered to be relatively high. ARDRAN (1970) reports the exposure at the skin to average 21.4 R during fluoroscopy plus 2.5 R during subsequent cineangiography. The effective areas varied from 16 to 390 cm^2 in the first case, and amounted from 95 to 390 cm^2 in the second. In our investigation, the radiation dose during the introduction and positioning of the catheters is not influenced by the measurement. According to BARON (1973), coronary angiography should be performed after the LV-pumping function has been established. For the ventriculographic part of the investigation, the administered dose may be estimated with the help of the dosage-rate *vs.* tube voltage data for various filtrations as published by WACHSMANN (1957). Considering its relative magnitude to the dose needed, the ventriculographic dose is not of prime importance.

IV. SUBTRACTION AS AN ASSISTANT TOOL

1. *Introduction*

The subtraction technique, as first described by ZIEDSES DES PLANTES in 1934, is a valuable adjunct in angiography when the contrast-filled cavities are obscured and overlapped by bone structures. The X-ray images are recorded on photographic film, a transparant negative of one picture is placed over a transparant positive of the other and subtraction is performed by exposing a third film through this combination.
This technique cancels, in theory at least, all picture elements common to the pair of radiographs. If a density has been added, usually in the form of an injected contrast medium, it will stand out with increased contrast, whereas unwanted structures are removed. Several authors have developed methods of subtraction which make use of various photographical procedures (CRITTENDEN,1966; RICE,1966), among which colour methods (WISE,1966). The applicability of subtraction in cineangiography had been shown earlier (VLASSENROOT,1961). The first to produce a subtracted image utilizing two television cameras and an inverting amplifier was HOLMAN (1963). Other systems, using electro-optical means to obtain electric signals which can be fed to a differential amplifier, have been given by ZIEDSES DES PLANTES (1966) and GROH (1967).

The flying-spot scanner principle as first used by BORGMANN (1956) for astronomical purposes, has successfully been applied to radiology by ROTH (1970). In videosubtraction, inequalities in the two camera chains show up in the result. To overcome this, use of only one TV chain and a memory for the videosignal was suggested by OOSTERKAMP, who developed a magnetic recording wheel (1961[b]). Recent developments in the field of magnetic disk recorders made further exploitation of this principle possible (HAAS,1969). The target of a silicon target storage tube, which stores the image as a positive or negative charge distribution depending on the energy of its electron beam, has also been used as an image memory for subtraction purposes in periodic fluoroscopic images (MISTRETTA,1973).

Subtraction has first been applied in neurology (brain circulation) and to renal examination, because movement artefacts are small in these cases. Recently, vacuum fixation has become available (VAN DIEREN,1973) as the method of choice for fastening the subject to the table, and has been used by us successfully.

Application to angiocardiography has mostly been limited to the demonstration of border movements (ZIEDSES DES PLANTES,1961; CHEN,1969). Respiration movement of the thoracic cage may be eliminated by holding the breath or by making pictures at a known phase of respiration when artificial respiration is used. Videosubtraction has found a useful application in fluoroscopy, *e.g.* selective angiography, since videodisks able to produce a stable still image came into use (HEINZE,1972). In angiography, the cavities to be studied are marked by a quantity of material with high absorption for X-ray radiation. Within limits, the validity of LAMBERT-BEER's law may be assumed (MOLDENHAUER,1972). The resulting videosignal may be regarded as proportional to the dose rate of X-ray radiation incident at the sensitive screen of the image intensifier. So, to obtain a signal which is a measure for the total amount of absorbing materials within a certain field of view, logarithmic conversion has to be applied (CHOW,1973). This conversion is performed in good approximation by the photographic film characteristics in photosubtraction, but has to be realized electronically in our case. JAEGER (1969) showed that the differential videosignal after conversion is proportional to the local contrast between regions with and without radiopaque medium. Moreover, unwanted structures, (ribs, diaphragm) have been removed from the image which corresponds to this differential videosignal.

If a quantitative evaluation of angiograms is to be performed, this signal should be taken as the basis for contour detection or videodensitometry.

Our objective is to evaluate the preprocessed videosignal for left ventricular volume measurements by semi-automatic methods (VAN WIJK VAN BRIEVINGH,1973[b]). It has already been observed that the human observer is able to discern some details in the subtraction results, which we cannot see in the original contrast picture. Moreover, if density profiles are to be used for reconstructing the area of an LV-slice from biplane projections (HEINTZEN,1974), using the subtraction result is indicated.

The same principle is used in digital form by TRENHOLM (1972) to find the local thickness of the left ventricle from a part of the TV-frame by computer. CHOW (1971) utilizes logarithmic conversion followed by subtraction to represent the radiation absorption in, and remove irrelevant background from, cineangiograms before a digital boundary detection algorithm is applied to the scanned images.

2. *Conversion of the Videosignal*

Beside asymmetrical magnification or distortion as described by BARRY (1963), image-intensifier television systems also exhibit a nonlinear behaviour in intensity, called shading. If a uniform intensity distribution is applied to the sensitive screen, the videosignal shows an amplitude which declines with the distance of the corresponding image points from the centre. As causes may be mentioned the curvature of the image intensifier input screen, and the greater thickness of the photosensitive layer in the middle compared with the border of the plumbicon (VAN DER POLDER,1967). In our system, shading amounted to about 13% from the centre to one quarter of both sides, if X-rays of 50 kV and 20 mA were applied with a layer of water of 15 cm thickness used as a scattering absorber. Electronic compensation[')] diminished this to the extent as depicted in Fig. 4.1; the third curve shows the shading signal, added to the cathode voltage of the plumbicon to achieve both horizontal and vertical correction. This signal consists of the superposition of a parabolic and a linear sawtooth.

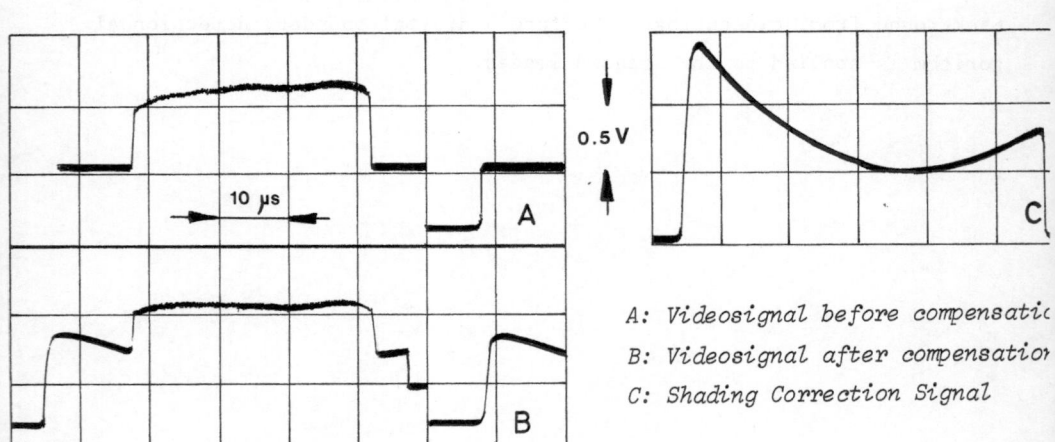

A: *Videosignal before compensation*
B: *Videosignal after compensation*
C: *Shading Correction Signal*

Fig. 4.1 Shading Correction of Imaging System

[')]Colorado Video Inc. type 608 Shading Generator.

The videosignals representing the images to be subtracted have to be converted logarithmically as mentioned in the preceding section. This procedure can be clarified by a simple model, in which a layer with thickness d of contrast medium with an absorption coefficient μ_2 is imbedded in a body with thickness D and an absorption coefficient μ_1. The difference ΔV of the logatithmically converted videosignals V_1 and V_2 is so a measure for $(\mu_1-\mu_2)d$, as illustrated in Fig. 4.2, based on JAEGER (1969). The contrast at the boundary of the regions appears to be approximately proportional to the differential videosignal ΔV.

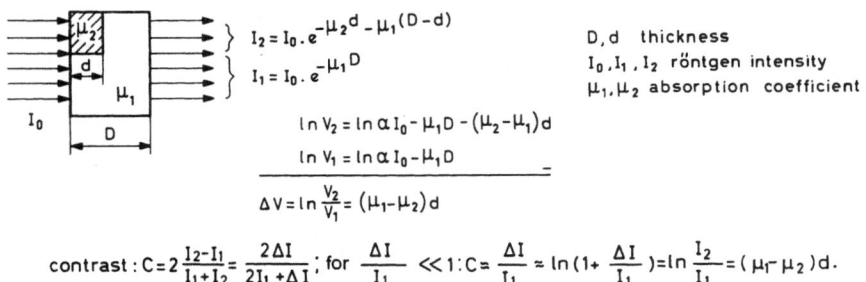

$$I_2 = I_0 . e^{-\mu_2 d - \mu_1(D-d)}$$

$$I_1 = I_0 . e^{-\mu_1 D}$$

D,d thickness
I_0, I_1, I_2 röntgen intensity
μ_1, μ_2 absorption coefficient

$$\ln V_2 = \ln \alpha I_0 - \mu_1 D - (\mu_2 - \mu_1)d$$

$$\ln V_1 = \ln \alpha I_0 - \mu_1 D$$

$$\Delta V = \ln \frac{V_2}{V_1} = (\mu_1 - \mu_2)d$$

$$\text{contrast}: C = 2\frac{I_2 - I_1}{I_1 + I_2} = \frac{2\Delta I}{2I_1 + \Delta I}; \text{ for } \frac{\Delta I}{I_1} \ll 1: C = \frac{\Delta I}{I_1} \approx \ln(1 + \frac{\Delta I}{I_1}) = \ln \frac{I_2}{I_1} = (\mu_1 - \mu_2)d.$$

Fig. 4.2 Absorption Model for Videosubtraction
The calculation shows that for this simplified model the contrast C is in approximation equal to the product of the thickness d of the contrast layer, and the difference of the mass absorption coefficients μ_1 and μ_2.

The logarithmic conversion of the part of the videosignal containing picture information is performed by two integrated units [')] in cascade, which feature a dynamic range of 30 dB and a rise time of 20-25 ns. As the noise level of the videosignal is of the order of 1 mV and the maximum image signal is about 1 V, not more than three decades are required, so a 90 dB total range is sufficient.

[')] Texas Instruments, type SN 76502

At the command of the central synchronization unit the parts of the signal consisting of the synchronization and blanking pulse pattern are removed by a videoswitch[')] which replaces them by a constant black level as zero reference. After conversion, the original synchronization pulse pattern is added again. The block-diagram is shown in Fig. 4.3.

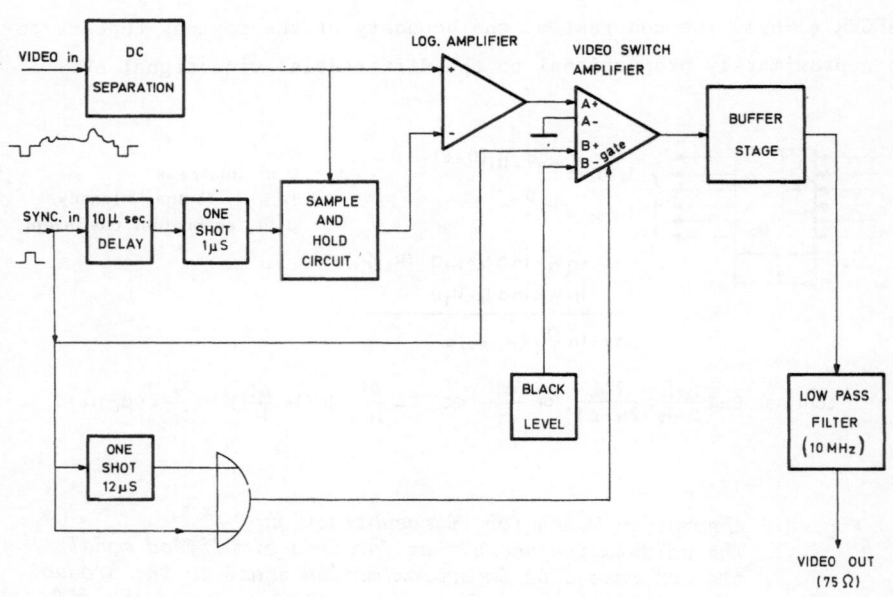

Fig. 4.3 Logarithmic Converter

[')] Motorola, MC 1445L

3. Procedure

The videodisk is equipped with two channels, on which different signals may be recorded simultaneously. The recording/reproducing heads of these channels, however, are coupled mechanically to one and the same mechanism, which is driven by a stepping motor. This means that the track numbers of the video-fields to be subtracted cannot be chosen independently. Thus, during the information registration phase great care must be taken that pictures of corresponding cardiac contraction phase with and without contrast medium are recorded at the same track numbers. In order to keep the electronical part of the disk system synchronized, the videosignal from the TV-chain is fed to both channels simultaneously. The channel on which the recording has to take place is then chosen by means of the remote disk control. The block-diagram of the registration phase is shown in Fig. 4.4.

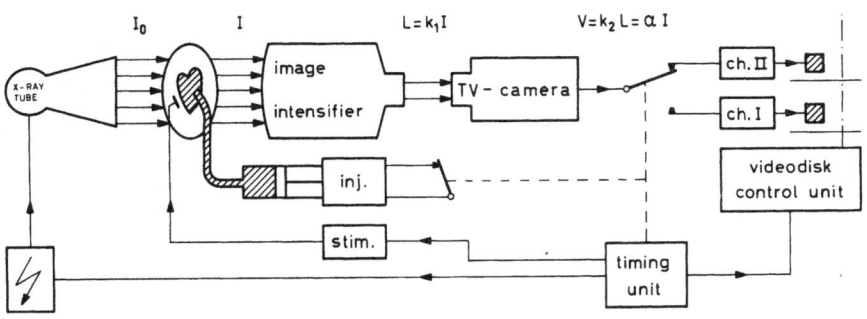

Fig. 4.4 Recording in Videosubtraction

At the command of the playback control, the signals recorded on corresponding tracks of both channels are continuously reproduced field-by-field for evaluation. The time base stability of the disk servo system corresponds to one picture element at the bandwidth given (100 ns at 4.3 MHz). Movement artefacts can be corrected to a small extent in vertical direction by inserting a 64 μs delay line as used in colour television into the leading channel. After logarithmic conversion, the signals are fed to the subtraction unit, the output signal of which is available for processing with a contour detection system or video-densitometer. The block diagram of Fig. 4.5 gives the evaluation part of the system.

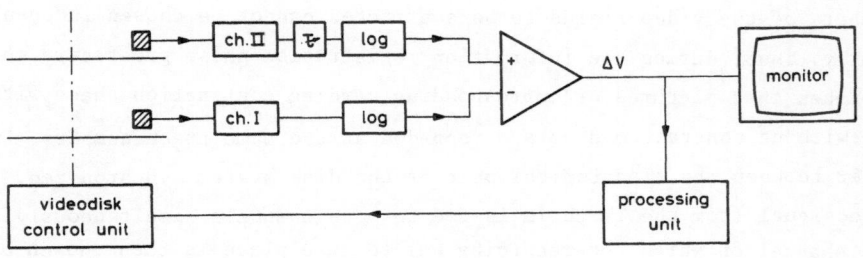

Fig. 4.5 Procedure of Videosubtraction

In the subtraction amplifier, removal of the synchronization pulse pattern and hard clamping are essential. The same principle as mentioned in the preceding section is applied, using the video-amplifier already described. The block-diagram is given in Fig. 4.6.

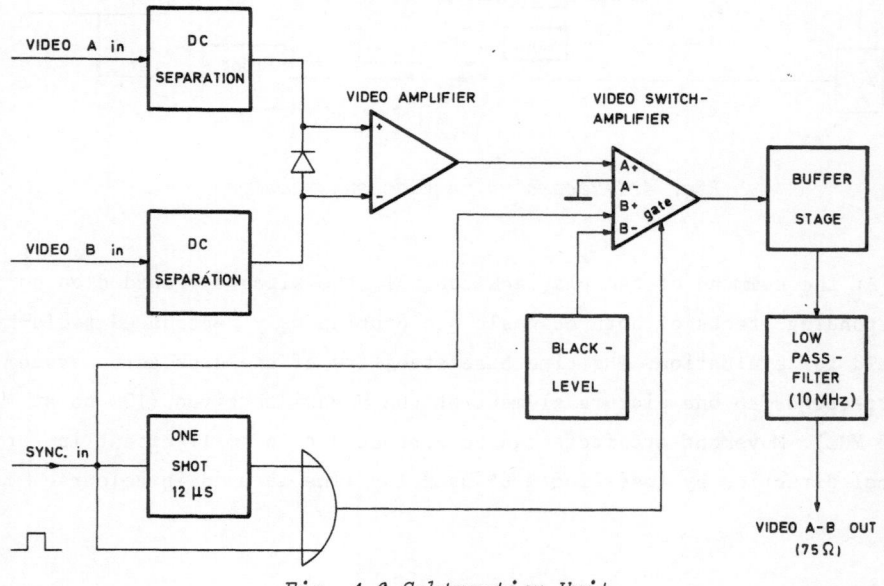

Fig. 4.6 Subtraction Unit

4. Example

Subtraction is used as a preprocessing procedure to facilitate contour detection, necessary for left ventricular volume determination. Non-relevant structures are removed so that the outline of the ventricular cavity, marked with radiopaque contrast medium, is more pronounced and can be drawn with a light-pen more easily. The results are shown in Fig. 4.7.
These pictures indicate, that the procedure described is a useful tool if quantitation of angiocardiography is to be achieved, although it requires a rather costly instrumentation and an intricate timing control of the measurement procedure.

(The hardware for handling of the videosignals has been developed by A.Richtering Blenken).

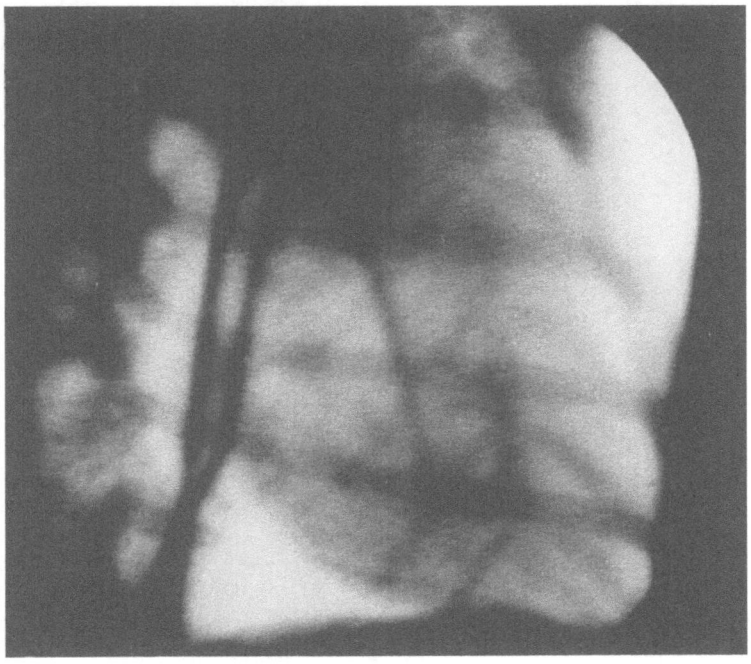

Fig. 4.7ᵃ End-diastolic picture of left ventricle without added contrast

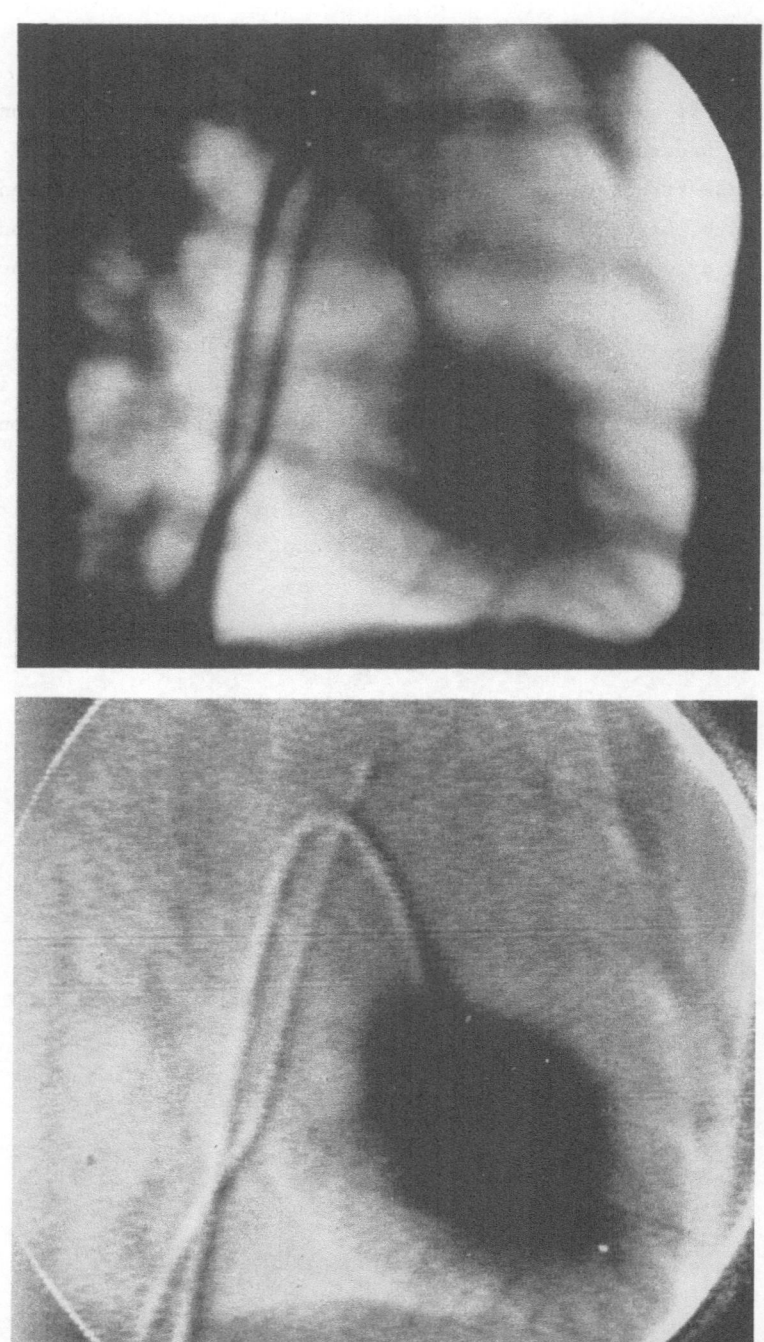

Fig. 4.7^b(top) Contrast-filled ventricle   Fig. 4.7^c(bottom) Subtraction Result

V. INTEGRATED INFORMATION RECORDING

1. *Introduction*

"The medical scene can be looked upon as a struggle to organize medical knowledge in such a way that it will be more useful to clinicians" (HALL, 1970). So an instrumental technique for diagnosis as developed here, should present its results in such a way, that they fit in the standardized basic data set used in the hospital (EPHRAIM,1974). Therefore, integrated recording of measurement results in combination with patient and administrative data was judged necessary. Coding has been chosen in accordance with the catheterization report form as used in the clinic. Recent technological developments made it possible to encode sufficient patient and administrative data together with measurement-results into the videosignal which carries the X-ray picture information, and record this combination on magnetic material. This is a logical extension of developments in cineangiocardiography, where extra information is recorded on the cinefilm by an optical path (MUDD,1960; STEWART,1969). It constitutes one of the functions of display systems in biomedical research (PERKINS,1971). Besides X-ray pictures, many measurements are taken during catheterization. Traditionally, the recording of these are made on several media, *e.g.* paper, oscilloscope screen or analog magnetic tape. In biplane cineangiocardiography, pairing of the corresponding pictures of the two films presents a time consuming problem, as well as sorting time markings on other recordings to collect the data in their proper time relationship. Furthermore, all registrations have to bear a patient identification, the date and other alphanumeric data. Even a semi-automatic protocol as described by REDLER (1972) still requires subsequent combination of radiographs and other data. With regard to the way of interpretation, this information can be divided into categories:

Morphologic information (X-ray pictures);
Analog data as a waveform (ECG, pressure curves);
Momentarily values of analog measurement results (LV and aortic pressure values, RR-intervals);
Digital numbers (parameters of the measurement system, frame numbers);
Alphanumeric information (patient identification, diagnostic data, date, name of physician, time).

As the X-ray pictures are already available in video format, devices were developed to encode this information into the corresponding TV-frame (VAN WIJK VAN BRIEVINGH,1974[b]).

This system compares favourably with other methods, one of which takes half of the monitor area if a TV-camera viewing an analog monitor screen is used. Moreover, it has a fairly small information capacity (OSYPKA, 1971[a],1071[b]).

Another principle encodes alphanumeric data produced by character generators into the TV-frame (KLEIN,1967; ZIMMERMANN,1971,1972; STEIGER, 1973), also at the cost of picture information.

A system based on coding in density levels at small image elements as described by JOHNSON (1974) offers a good capacity, but is only applicable together with a videodensitometer.

Since in general the outer vertical quarter parts of the field of view contain no details relevant to contour determination of the LV-shadow, these regions may be used for other purposes. Firstly, this provides the possibility to combine in one frame both views of the biplane X-ray system. This may be performed rather easily by introducing suitable time delays into the line synchronization pulse pattern (OSYPKA,1971[a]). With the "Vidicor" (HEMELAAR, internal report M 89), momentarily-retrospective curves of the most recent five seconds of two signals (ECG and LV-pressure) as well as a time scale and two event marking channels are presented in vertical bands at the left and middle of the frame. From these curves visual interpretation of the preceding heart-beats becomes possible.

The "Anacor" (COENEN, internal report M 101) encodes the values of up to four analog signals, sampled at the moment of the X-ray flash, into time intervals between pulse pairs on selected lines of the videoframe. Besides, the time elapsed since the last ED-pulse (R-wave) is also encoded with a resolution of 2 milliseconds. The principle has been chosen in such a way, that the video-computer interface is able to transfer these data directly. By means of the "Digicor" (DE KRIJGER, internal report 051560-28,1973,22), up to 800 alphanumeric characters are encoded as binary words into the first and last 32 lines of each videoframe. These lines are not visually displayed on the monitor. The corresponding characters may be displayed on a second TV-monitor simultaneously or on the same screen if the other picture is switched off.

The Digicor is compatible with the computer as the ASCII (teletype) code is used. A registration "form" may be introduced into its digital memory by papertape, the administrative and other data can be typed in with a teletype. During the measurement, the text may be changed manually or automatically (frame numbering, time and date from a digital clock).

Thus, patient data and measurement parameters are recorded simultaneously with the measured data on the same medium (videotaperecorder or disk) as shown in Fig. 5.1. High information density and flexibility of use favours this solution to other methods described.

For X-ray pictures in which the limited bandwidth of the TV-frames offers no constraint to the spatial resolution, files on videotape, perhaps to be kept with the audiovisual department of the hospital, is an attractive possibility (RECOURT,1972).

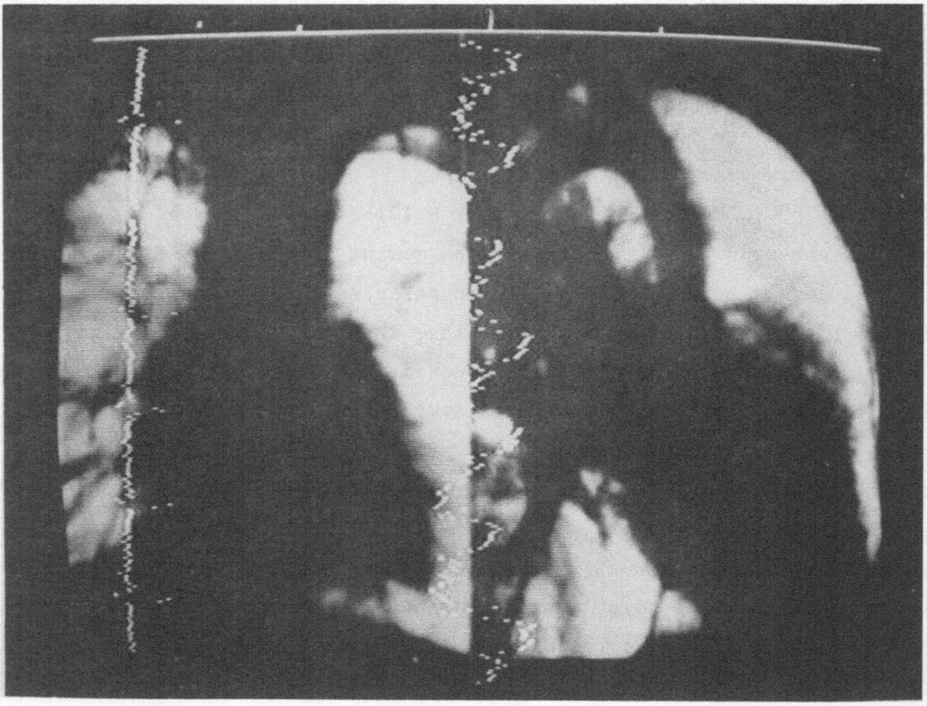

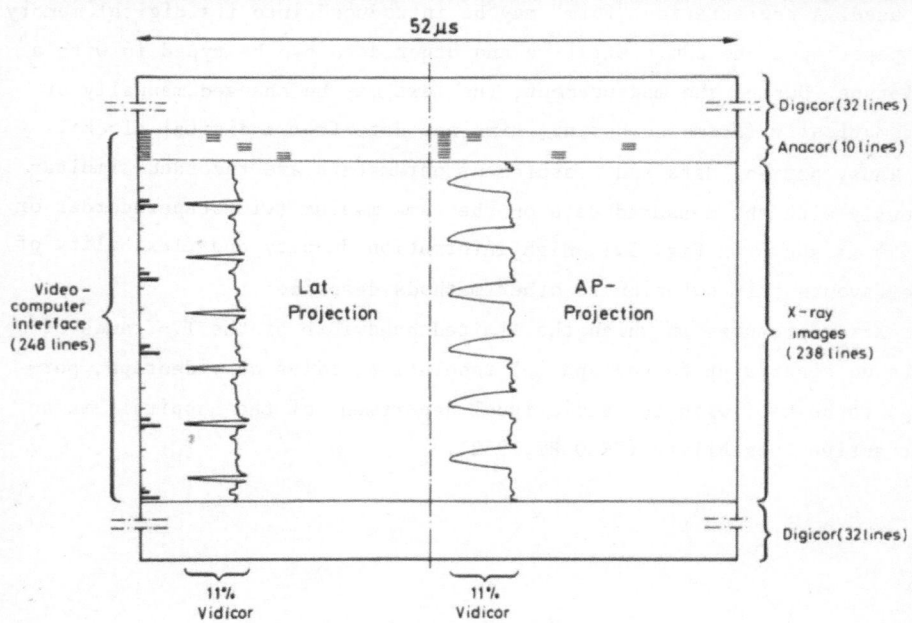

Fig. 5.1 Integrated Information Recording
Top: Monitor picture.
Bottom: Schematic.

2. *Vidicor*

To judge the state of contraction of a ventricle as exactly as possible, the cardiologist has to supplement his visual interpretation of the vi-deo-angiocardiogram with ECG and pressure signals (GEBAUER,1965). Moreover, the moment and duration of the contrast medium injections are essential in relation to these data.

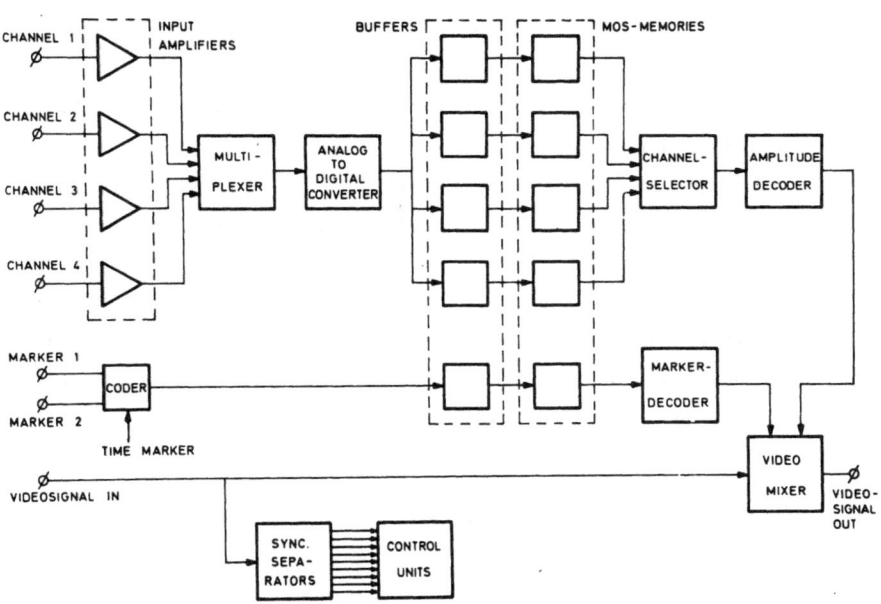

Fig. 5.2 Vidicor

The "Vidicor", the block diagram of which is shown in Fig. 5.2, presents in visual form the most recent 5.1 seconds of up to 4 signals, sampled at 64 levels, with a frequency of 300 Hz, as well as a time reference and two event markings. For this purpose, about 11% of the net width of the monitor picture is reserved for each data channel.
Because of the low price per bit and the relatively simple control, MOS static shift registers of 512 sections each are used as memory elements.

The signals are multiplexed to the A/D converter. The corresponding samples are retained in 6-bit latches. After insertion of the sample values into the shift registers, their contents are clocked round, while the decoded output is converted into an image point on the relevant TV line. The control unit supplies programming pulses to the multiplexer, the A/D converter and the latches, as well as to the signal selector, in synchronism with the TV-frame. A "freezing" mode is available.

The data channels have a cut-off frequency of 800 Hz; the input amplifier gain of 1 to 50 may be continuously adjusted, a DC offset from -5 to +5 V may be compensated. Input voltages from 100 mV to 5 V peak-to-peak superimposed on a DC level may thus be accepted. The marking channels give an indication if a trigger level, adjustable from -5 to +5 V, is surpassed. The memory contents may be shifted each frame or each field, in order to achieve a stable real-time presentation. (HEMELAAR, internal report M89).

This preludes on the possibility of recording one frame instead of one field per revolution of the videodisk. As soon as the manufacturer can apply this modification, the sampling frequency of our system can be doubled to 50 images per second, thus overcoming one of its main limitations.

3. Anacor

As stated in Chapter I, the LVV as calculated frame-by-frame has to be
related to other quantities measured, *e.g.* the LV-pressure to construct
pressure-volume loops (HEINTZEN,1971[e]), or the duration of the preceding
RR-intervals. To simplify the evaluation procedure, it is desirable to
use the same interface for this purpose as is coupled to the contour
memory.

Coding of analog values as "bars" in the TV-picture has been described
as an adjunct to videodensitometric methods (HEINTZEN,1971[b]), the procedure of redrawing these "controlled windows" with a light-pen, however, introduces an avoidable extra error.

The coding and recording of the LV-contour as sampled per TV-line
will be described in detail in section VIII-2. The "Anacor" converts
analog signal values to time intervals between pulse pairs, and encodes
the corresponding pulses into the videosignal. The block-diagram of the
Anacor input part is shown in Fig. 5.3. (COENEN, internal report M 101).

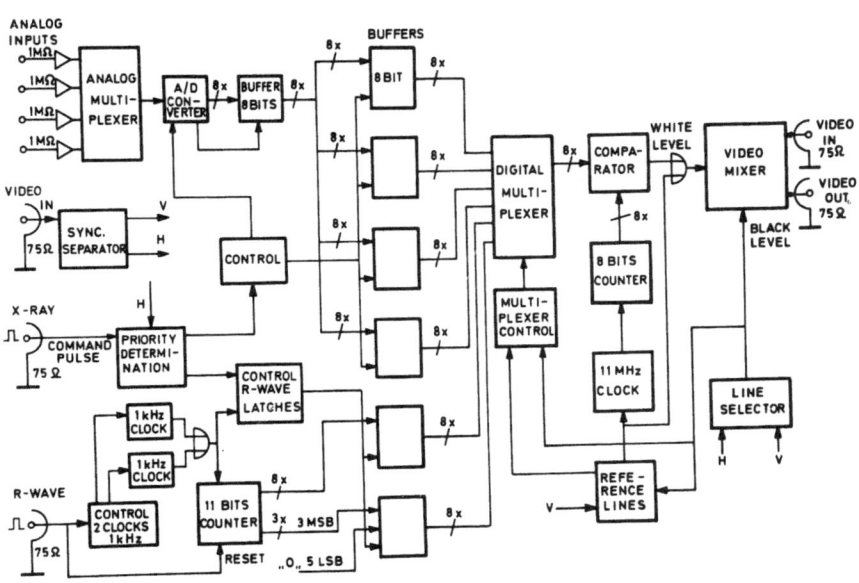

Fig. 5.3 Anacor Input Section

Up to 4 analog signals are sampled at the moment of the X-ray flashes as well as the time elapsed since the most recent R-wave of the ECG. These quantities are retained in 8-bit latches, the outputs of which are multiplexed at the command of pulses in synchronism with the TV-synchronization pattern. For encoding into the TV frame, 10 lines are reserved, so that two channels can be situated on three successive lines; the 10th line is switched white in its entirety for visual indication. As a resolution of 1 ms is required in the RR-interval measurement, two channels are used for the registration of the elapsed time. This time is measured with two 1 kHz clocks, each of which is started in an alternating mode upon occurence of each R-wave. The corresponding contents of an 11-bit counter are fed to two 8-bit latches, the second one of which contains the three most significant bits only. This implies, that the elapsed time has to be decoded by software. A comparator gives a marking signal, to be recorded in the videosignal as a white image point, each time the contents of an 8-bit counter are equal to the contents of the corresponding latch, thus encoding the relevant signal samples into distances between pulses on the pertinent TV-lines. These pulses are to be transferred automatically to the digital contour memory during the off-line evaluation procedure.

4. *Digicor*

Some measurement results or parameters of the system become available
in numerical form. Bookkeeping of the measurement (frame and injection
numbers) delivers results in digital form. Patient and administrative
data are given alphanumerically. Integrated recording of these data in
a form compatible with the basic data set to be used for medical registration is required as stated in section V-1.
It is possible to make use of the field blanking period of the television signal, as common in communication TV for so-called "insertion signals" on the lines 16 and 329 (HUTT,1973). Owing to the finite dimension
of the recording head in magnetic tape and disk recorders, a number
of lines near the field synchronization pulse cannot be used because of
"drop-out". The method described by OSYPKA (1971[a]) uses one data channel
(digital counter or A/D converter) with 8 bits per field per TV-line
and therefore has a limited capacity.

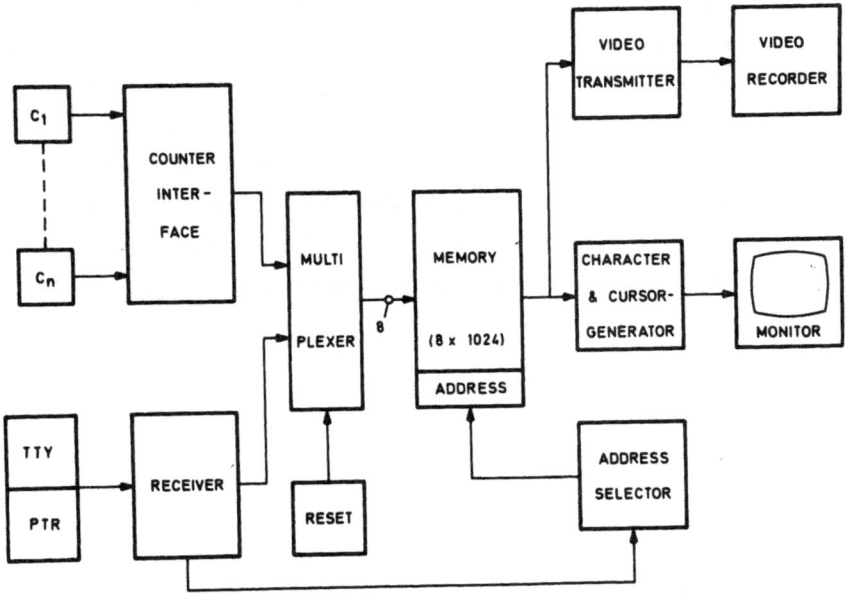

Fig. 5.4 Digicor Input Section

For our purpose, the "Digicor" has been developed. The block-diagram of the input part of it is given in Fig. 5.4. It can comprise a message of 800 alphanumeric characters, structured in 25 lines of 32 characters each. To facilitate computer handling, a "form" has been designed so that the nature of parts of the message is coupled to the position of the corresponding characters within the array. This form can be intro- duced by papertape. The 8-bits binary words corresponding to the charac- ters of the form text contain an identification bit, in order to prevent them from being overwritten by teletype during the filling-out of the form. A cursor indicates automatically the first free character position to be used. During the write-in mode the characters are displayed on the TV-screen, and the corresponding binary words are retained in eight 1024-bit MOS dynamic random access memories[1], which are refreshed every 16×64 µs ≈ 11 ms at the moments of occurence of line synchroniza- tion pulses. The first 32 characters are used for the contents of coun- ters or other devices giving their output in digital form A multiplexer selects the access to the memory. A line selector controls the 25 line periods at the beginning and end of each frame during which the message is encoded. The resulting binary videosignal, contains a parity bit and three synchronization bits. The code used requires a bandwidth of 3.25 MHz. This videosignal is mixed with the signals from the other devices as described in the preceding section (DE KRIJGER, internal report). An example of the binary coded as well as of the alphanumerical message, combined into one picture for illustration purposes, is given in Fig. 5.5.

---

[1] INTEL RAM 1103

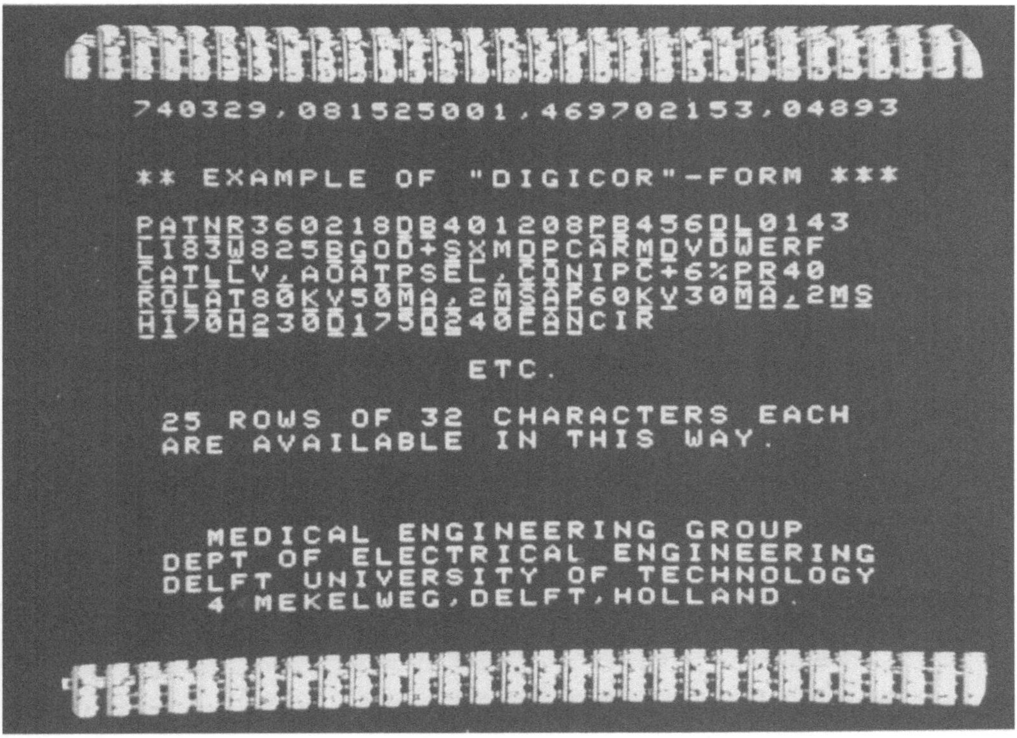

Fig. 5.5 Example of Digicor Recording and Presentation
The bands at the top and at the bottom of the picture show
the binary code, divided into words which appear as groups
of dots.
The middle part gives the alphanumeric representation of the
message. This text is the same as would be printed on tele-
type or read into the computer.

5. *Magnetic Recording of the Videosignal*

The videosignal, containing all relevant information as described before, is recorded on one track of a videodisk[') and represents one
sample in the measuring process. The disk, however, can only contain
2 x 600 fields, and thus serves as an intermediate registration medium.
Although some aspects have been studied (VAN DER PADT, internal report
M 104), the development of a "Video-Tapery" as archives on magnetic
material, falls outside the scope of this thesis. Videotaperecorders to
be used in such a system should meet severe requirements as to time base
stability (WHITE, 1972). Within a department, a videodisk equipped with
peripheral control should be time-shared between the angiography and
other rooms (GEBAUER, 1965). The videotape editing facility should be
centralized, preferably at the Audiovisual Department. So, a network
of image recording and reproducing units, interconnected by a suitable
transmission system could be set up, servicing many Departments and
reducing cost and filing space.

[') AMPEX MD 400

VI. THE GEOMETRIC MODEL

1. *Introduction*

As mentioned in section II-1, the X-ray installation as a measurement
tool was already made use of in the beginning of this century. Some
methods in use nowadays for the determination of intraventricular volume
originate from those applied to total heart volume measurement. Since
the introduction of the orthodiagraphic projection method by MORITZ
(1900), clinicians have looked for a basis to compare the size of hearts
in a quantitative way. GEIGEL (1914) has often been criticized for the
simplicity of the ball model he suggested, although in his article he
admits several times that this is not a geometrical approximation but
only a measure to be used in comparative studies. From the volume
$V = 4F^{\frac{3}{2}}/3\sqrt{\pi}$, in which formula F equals the planimetered area of the
heart shadow, he derived a "reduced heart quotient" by omitting the
numerical factor and dividing by body weight (normal values are 15-23).
Basing himself on dimensional considerations, ROHRER (1916) gave several
formulae for the determination of body cavity volumes from linear or
area measurements. Depending on the choice, different numerical constants were applied; these factors are the least dependent on shape if
as many area measures as possible are used. From parallel projections

in two perpendicular directions (sagittal and transversal) the shadow
area F and largest diameter L were determined respectively, and next
the cardiac volume was calculated with V = 0.63 F.L. The constant chosen
was the average value of the factor which may be calculated in similar
expressions for a sphere (0.66) and a paraboloid (0.59); it proved to
correspond excellently with experiments with a heart model which gave
the value 0.62.

BARDEEN (1918) described a method for determination of F and L with
teleradiography by means of a known displacement of the X-ray tube.
In 1932, KAHLSTORF introduced the ellipsoid as a geometric model for
the heart. He showed, that independent of the direction of its axes
relative to the plane of (parallel) projection, the volume may be found
from V = 2/3 F L , in which F and L are defined as above. JONSELL (1939)
suggested to obviate planimetry by the assumption that the heart shadow
is an ellipse, the area of which may be determined from its long and
short axis lengths directly. He related the heart volume thus found
with the body surface area as determined with help of the body height
and weight according to the formula given by DU BOIS (1927). The use of
the body surface area is based on considerations of metabolism and yields
a heart volume index. This seems to be a better basis than the index
based on heart silhouette diameter only as described by UNGERLEIDER
(1939). Cardiac volume determination based on biplane projections and a
slice method has been described by LARSSON (1948). Hereby, SIMPSON's
rule is applied to the addition of the disk volumes expressed by the
product of sets of diameters in the shadow contours parallel to the
X-ray beam. The author rejected an alternative method in which the shape
of the disks had been accounted for by a general factor, because of the
tedium and time cost of calculations.

KJELLBERG (1951), tested the accuracy of an alternative method, namely
an ellipsoid for which V = f a b c with a and b the diameters, corrected
for magnification of the AP-projection, and c the greatest corrected
diameter of the lateral view. The factor f, which in the case of an
ellipsoid would have equalled $\pi/6$, was determined experimentally as a
variable c^2/ab, but proved statistically to be allowed for by a constant

dependent on heart shape. The slice method has been put into practice
by DUHAMEL (1954) with slices obtained by tomography.

GEBHARDT (1957) used one picture to determine the depth of the heart and
seven planigraphic pictures for area contour demonstration. The model
used by him for volume calculation consisted of a set of seven cylinders,
having a cone in the front and at the back. The height of the components
was determined from a lateral view.

FONTANILLE (1960) devised a nomogram for calculating the cardiac volume
according to $V = f \ a \ b \ c$. with $f = 0.40$ including the magnification correction. A comparative study of the precision of the models in use with
help of a set of paraffin casts has been published by GEBHARDT (1969),
who arrived at the conclusion that his own method was the best. As lately
as 1965, EVANS investigated the errors of the ellipsoid-approximation
technique by comparison with post-mortem hearts. He found the biggest
potential error to be observer variation in making the axis measurements
from the X-ray films.

As will be shown in the next section, many methods used in LVV-determination have been derived from the principles mentioned above.

2. Survey of Models

Until the nineteen-fifties, modeling had been applied mainly to the total heart, rather than to specific chambers. Cineangiographic methods have been used by RUSHMER (1951[a];1951[b]) to study the configuration of the ventricular chambers and the mechanics of ventricular contraction in dogs. Besides conclusions on the functional anatomy (1953) this author computed the ventricular area, which was taken to be an index of volume, and plotted it as a function of time. From the observations of the configuration, the left ventricle was approximated by a thick-walled cylinder with a cone on top.

In similar experiments in which the ECG had been included, GRIBBE (1958) showed, that the isometric contraction starts at the moment, when the LV has reached its greatest volume. This moment proved to coincide reasonably with the peak of the R-wave. In 1959, the same author described the LV-cavity as an ellipsoid. Based on the observation that the diameters in left and right oblique projection were in constant proportion with a factor 0.85; the volume may be calculated from only one projection:

$$V = 0.85 \; \frac{\pi}{6} \; D_1^2 \; L \; \ldots \ldots \ldots \ldots \ldots \ldots \ldots \ldots \ldots \quad (6.1)$$

This formula still has to be corrected multiplicatively for projection magnification and additively by the volume of the *trabeculae carneae* and the papillary muscles.

CHAPMAN in 1958 introduced his famous method in which the LVV is computed as a summation of elementary volumes, according to SIMPSON's rule. Thereby, the slices are described as elliptic cylinders. The diameters from the LV-shadow contours in biplane cineangiograms are taken as the axes, so

$$V = \frac{\pi}{3} \; (\underset{odd}{\Sigma} \; x_i \; y_i + \tfrac{1}{2} \underset{even}{\Sigma} \; x_j \; y_j) \; \ldots \ldots \ldots \ldots \ldots \quad (6.2)$$

in which h equals the height of the slices (in the order of 1 mm) and x and y are the respective diameters in the LAO and RAO projections.

The time-consuming calculations became feasible in practice after the introduction of digital computers in this field; an optical contour scanner system as described by BAKER (1961) or standard computer scanner sheets according to GOERKE (1967) came into use as input media.

In 1960, after a preliminary report in 1956, DODGE published several methods for the calculation of LVV from biplane angiocardiograms, the usefulness and limitations of which were established in 1966 by the same author.

Three of these methods use a general ellipsoid as the geometric model, for which the volume

$$V = \frac{\pi}{6} L \, D_1 \, D_2 \quad \ldots \ldots \ldots \ldots \ldots \ldots \ldots \quad (6.3)$$

L being the major axis, and D_1, D_2 the minor axes.

The long axis of the ellipsoid may be chosen to correspond with the apex to mid-aortic valve length as computed from the projections of the corresponding points or the longest measured image length in either projection, corrected for distortion due to nonparallel X-rays. The minor axes may be taken to be the corrected maximum diameters perpendicular to the long axis or the apex to mid-mitral valve line ("three measured length method") or computed as the corrected minor axes of the equivalent ellipses in both projections

$$D_{1,2} = \frac{4}{\pi} \frac{A_{1,2}}{L} \quad \ldots \ldots \ldots \ldots \ldots \ldots \ldots \quad (6.4)$$

in which $A_{1,2}$ are the planimetered areas of the LV shadow contours ("area-length method").

Contrary to the findings in dogs, DODGE (1966) states that in patients the two minor diameters of the left ventricular chamber do not differ significantly from one another, so single-plane angiocardiograms might be used as well.

The "area product method", as suggested by CHAPMAN (1958), makes use of the planimetered areas only; the empirical relations between the LVV and the product of the areas have been established by this author.

DODGE (1960) calculated for human subjects:

$$\log V = 0.7762 \log (A_1 A_2) - 0.405 \text{ ml} \quad \ldots \ldots \ldots \ldots \quad (6.5)$$

From comparisons with post-mortem hearts, the same author computed regression corrections for the biplane methods to be applied in man:

Area-length method : $V_{true} = 0.928 V_{calc.} - 3.8 \text{ ml}$ . . . . . (6.6)
SIMPSON's rule method: $V_{true} = 0.849 V_{calc.} - 3.9 \text{ ml}$ . . . . . (6.7)

For the use of single plane angiocardiograms in man, SANDLER (1968) computed the following regression equations:

Longest measured length in A-P projection L_A *vs* spatial length L:
$L_A = 0.987 L - 0.02 \text{ cm}$ . . . . (6.8)
Ventricular volume as calculated from A-P films with the area length
method
$$V_A = \frac{\pi}{6} L_A D_A^2 \quad \ldots \ldots \ldots \ldots \ldots \ldots \ldots \ldots \quad (6.9)$$
vs biplane area-length volumes, corrected with the above-mentioned
regression formula;
$V = 0.951 V_A - 3.0 \text{ ml}$ . . . . (6.10)

Meanwhile, the development of relatively fast (6 pairs of images per
second) biplane film changers had led ARVIDSSON to angiocardiographic
LAV-determination from large size pictures (1957). An ellipsoid model
as used for the left atrium in mitral disease has been used in modified
form by this author for LVV-measurements (1961). In true anterio-poste-
rior (A-P), and lateral projections, the LV-shadows are each described
by two half ellipses, the ventricular cavity being approximated by two
semi-ellipsoids. The long axis of the total body is determined from the
orthogonal projections L_1 and L_2, after correction for the projection
magnification with factors f_1 and f_2, corresponding with the position
of the approximate center of the ellipsoid.
The maximum diameters, D_1 and D_2, perpendicular to this long axis, may

also be readily determined and used for calculation of the lower semi-ellipsoid. The point between the mitral and aortic orifices is usually obtained directly in the AP-projection. It may be transferred to the lateral shadow because it must lie at the same horizontal level.
The lower border of the left atrium may be used as a reference.
The projections of the major axis are constructed by finding the centre point on the transverse axis and drawing the line from the apex out to this centre point. The spatial length is calculated with the assistance of the lengths of the two projections and the angle β formed by the axis projection with the horizontal plane in the AP- projection.
Thus, the left ventricular volume is found to be

$$V = \frac{\Pi}{6} \frac{D_1}{f_1} \frac{D_2}{f_2} \sqrt{\frac{L_1^2 \cos^2\beta}{f_1^2} + \frac{L_2^2}{f_2^2}} \quad \ldots \ldots \ldots \ldots \ldots \ldots \quad (6.11)$$

as described by ARVIDSSON (1966). In 1967, the same author discussed the continuous change in geometrical magnification along the long axis of the ventricular ellipsoid, but did not give a practical solution to this problem.

After several of the models described above had been in use for some years, their accuracy could be determined on a statistical basis.
SANMARCO (1966) as well as DAVILA (1966[b]) performed this with the help of left-ventricular casts, the true volume of which could be measured accurately by water displacement. All models tended to overestimate this true volume systematically, so correction by a regression equation is mandatory. The two most important factors for the overestimation are the volume occupied by the papillary muscles, the *trabeculae carneae*, and the *chordae tendinae*, and the degree of misfit between the model and the true shape of the ventricle.
GREENE (1967) states that a simple monoplane method can be obtained with an ellipsoid of revolution as a model. The major axis, L, is drawn from the apex to the atrio-ventricular intersection point and the minor axis is determined by the middleperpendicular thereof.
Other suggestions for simplification of techniques in this field have been given by HERMANN (1968).

		A-P proj (magn factor f_1)	lat proj (magn factor f_2)	

| 1 | DODGE (1956 - 1960) $$V_{calc} = \frac{\pi}{6} \cdot L \cdot D_1 \cdot D_2$$ $$V_{true} = 0.928 \, V_{calc} - 3.8 \text{ ml.}$$ | D_1 A_1 | A_2 D_2 — equivalent ellipses — | $A_{1,2}$ planimetered $D_{1,2} = \frac{4}{\pi} \cdot \frac{A_{1,2}}{L}$ end-points of L, D_1, D_2 corrected for projection |

| 2 | ARVIDSSON (1957) $$V = \frac{\pi}{6} \cdot \frac{D_1}{f_1} \cdot \frac{D_2}{f_2} \sqrt{\frac{L_1^2 \cos^2\beta}{f_1^2} + \frac{L_2^2}{f_2^2}}$$ | D_1 L_1 | β D_2 L_2 | $D_{1,2}$ maximum diameters perpendicular to $L_{1,2}$ |

| 3 | CHAPMAN (1958) $$\log V = 0.7762 \log(A_1 \cdot A_2) - 4.05 \text{ ml}$$ (regression by DODGE, 1960) | A_1 | A_2 | $A_{1,2}$ planimetered |

| 4 | CHAPMAN (1958) $$V_{calc} = \frac{\pi}{3} h \left(\sum_{odd} x_i y_i + \frac{1}{2} \sum_{even} x_i y_i \right)$$ $$V_{true} = 0.849 \, V_{calc} - 3.9 \text{ ml.}$$ (regression by DODGE, 1960) | x_i | y_i | |

| 5 | GREENE (1967) $$V = \frac{\pi}{6} \cdot \frac{L \cdot D^2}{f_1^3}$$ | L D | | D = length of middleperpendicular to L |

| 6 | SANDLER (1968) $$V_A = \frac{\pi}{6} \cdot L_A \cdot D_A^2$$ $$L_A = 0.987 \, L - 0.02 \text{ cm}$$ $$V = 0.951 \, V_A - 3.0 \text{ ml.}$$ | L_A A D_A | | A planimetered, L = longest measured length, $D_A = \frac{4}{\pi} \cdot \frac{A}{L_A}$ |

| 7 | VAN WIJK VAN BRIEVINGH (1973) $$V = \frac{h}{3} \left[\sum_{odd} a_i(\beta, \gamma, \psi) \frac{x_i y_i}{f_{1_i} f_{2_i}} + \frac{1}{2} \sum_{even} a_i(\beta, \gamma, \psi) \frac{x_i y_i}{f_{1_i} f_{2_i}} \right]$$ | x_i β | y_i γ | $h = \frac{L}{n}$; L = true spatial length $a_i(\beta, \gamma, \psi)$ from casts |

Fig. 6.1 Survey of Geometric Models

Diagrams of the models discussed above are given in Fig. 6.1.

Several of the above-mentioned investigators specify the positioning of their subjects relative to the X-ray installation. GRIBBE (1959) used a lead marker to indicate the position of the apex as determined by palpation on the chest wall. BENTIVOGLIO (1972), however, criticizes heavily those authors who do not provide these data. In his experiments, he compares angiograms *in vivo* and of casts of the same dogs in exactly the same position. To this end, long needles are placed through the thorax and the ventricle which has to be filled with cast material after the animal has been sacrificed. The needle positions are fixed relative to the installation by means of styrofoam blocks which are used again when the casts' shadows are pictured. A coordinate reference system relative to the dog's body is given, and regression formulae for some of the geometric models are presented. The study indicates that the average degree of right-anterior oblique (RAO) rotation which is necessary to place the longitudinal axis of the LV on or near the plane normal to the oncoming X-rays amounts to about 67°. The coordinate axes have been chosen in partial agreement with the convention used in electro and vectorcardiography.

In the publications of SANMARCO (1966) and DAVILA (1966[b]) slices of LV-casts are shown, demonstrating the irregular shape of the ventricular cavity, especially the "impressions" made by the papillary muscles and the *trabeculae carneae*. A geometric model based on LV-cast slices has been proposed (VAN WIJK VAN BRIEVINGH,1973[a],1974[a]), and will be explained in the following sections. It has been developed independent of the correction factor method as described by SANTAMORE (1973) for monoplane pictures.

3. *Preparation of Casts*

Determination of the volume of irregularly shaped bodies by water displacement goes back to ARCHIMEDES OF SYRACUSE (287-212 BC); application of this principle to bees wax' casts of ventricular cavities was reported by HALES in 1733. A method for radiological measurement of the total heart's volume and shape in living subjects has been attempted by PALMIERI (1920;1929). He developed a technique in which a model was continuously adjusted to the heart shadows of the patient ("Radioplastic"). The same principle was used by TAKAHASHI as recent as in 1954 under the name of "Solidography". Evidently this involves much expenditure of time and irradiation to the patient. Cutting of styrofoam blocks according to the LV-contours drawn on biplane angiographic films has been performed by CARLSSON (1966). He established a close correspondance of the styrofoam model weight to the weight of silicone ventricular casts, for the left as well as for the right ventricular cavity. The use of casts has long been known to anatomists, but the development of two-component plastics made possible the corrosion casting technique which is extensively used in the investigation of the vascular system (BUGGE,1963). Requirements for these plastics are, a regulable viscosity, sufficient working time after combining the two components, inmiscibility with water, minimal shrinkage and resistibility to the corroding agents used to do away with the structures around the injected cavities.
Evidently, radiopaqueness is also of importance for our purpose. In collaboration with the preparation division of the Department of Anatomy, Medical Faculty of the University of Utrecht [), a suitable technique for preparation of ventricular casts was introduced in the Laboratory for Experimental Cardiology. In a first attempt, read-lead was used as an additive to obtain greater radiopacity. During the harding, however, unmixing took place. In the second set of casts made, a stabilizer called "Irgastab 17M" and containing tin as the X-ray contrast medium,

---

[) Thanks are due to H. Kemperman for his assistance.

proved a good additive['], (an organo-dibuthyl-tin mercaptid).

It is of importance to obtain a set of casts of ventricles in a known contractile state. Techniques for rapid fixation in systole or diastole under known haemodynamic conditions have been described by ROSS (1967) who applied the fixative glutaraldehyde to an analysis of the geometry of the ventricular cavity, its muscular walls, and the papillary muscles. This agent has been proved not to produce contracture of isolated heart muscle. The state of contraction of the hearts to be fixated was determined by this author based on the LV-pressure, the ECG, as well as on the configuration of the ventricular cavity. The casts were made by filling the excised heart with liquid, room temperature vulcanizing, silicone rubber. This method may be criticed, as thoracotomy is known to produce shrinkage of the heart (RUSHMER,1954). Therefore, the use of catheterization procedures to inject an arresting agent into the left coronary artery as described by BENTIVOGLIO (1972) has been preferred by us. In dogs to be sacrificed, videoangiocardiograms have been recorded on the videodisk prior to the fixation. The frame representing the contractile state chosen, has been selected by frame-by-frame playback and watching the ECG and LV-pressure curves as displayed by the "Vidicor", described in section V-2. The LV-contour was then copied with an ink pencil on the TV-monitor window. After arresting the heart as described above, the mixture of two-component plastic["] with the Irgastab contrast medium was injected until the shadow borders coincided with the contour drawn previously. After harding overnight the heart was excised. Next, erosion of the cardiac muscle by boiling the preparation in potassium hydroxyde was performed and the stumps at the aortic and mitral valves were removed. The volume was determined by water displacement. According to marks indicating the end-points of the axis of the ventricular cavity,

---

[']Obtained from A.E.M. Keyzers, Department of Physical Chemistry, Delft University of Technology, Manufacturer: Ciba-Geigi.

["]Brand:Plexigum; Type M356

and the midline over the septal part, the casts could be placed in the optical shadowing device to be described in the next section and in specially made matrices to embed them in transparant epoxy resin[']. The length having been divided into 20 equal parts, the block was sawn into slices perpendicular to the axis, thus obtaining the cross-sections at equidistant points. From these cross-sections, shown in Fig. 6.2 measurements of shape and area of the slices could be made for the construction of our geometric model. It is recognized that the active contractile state and the contracture obtained by the procedure above are different in principle. In practice, however, we believe that the results obtained are as close as possible to the physiologic reality (YANG, 1972). The relation between the shadows obtained in angiocardiography and the anatomical details of the casts could be established on the basis of illustrations in an article of RAPHAEL (1974). Characteristic points in the LV-shadow projections have been indicated as a basis for contour definition by BESSE (1974).

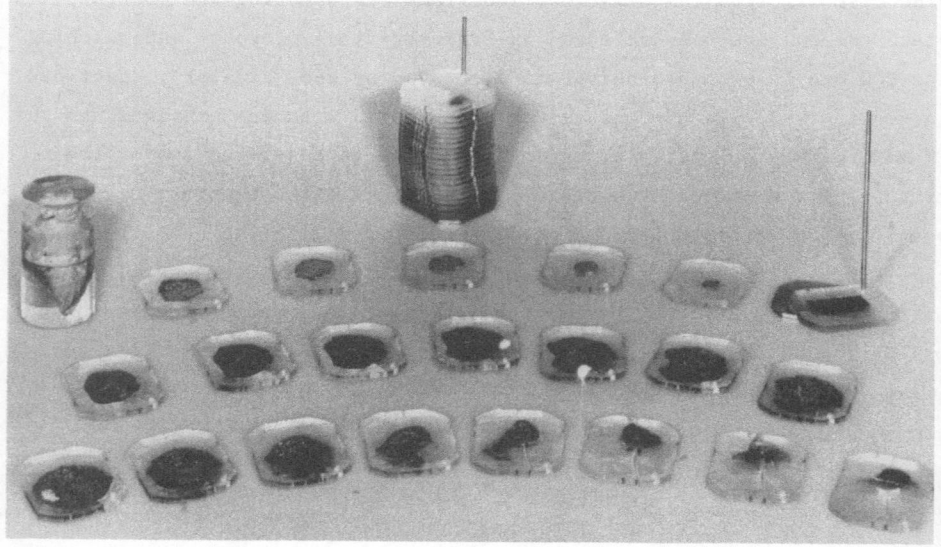

Fig. 6.2 Example of Ventricular Casts

[']Brand:Romar-Voss, Type:6TS

4. Index of Irregularity

The contrast shadows in biplane projections contain the primary information available on the ventricle under study. This means that a geometric model has to be assumed, according to which the volume is calculated. As the shape of the ventricle is irregular, this model must bear a relationship to the anatomic reality which is as close as possible. Video techniques offer the feature to digitize the LV-contours by the TV-scanning lines. Many times, the model according to Chapman (1958) is used with slices corresponding to these lines. The only stereometric body giving elliptical cross-sections irrespective of the direction of intersection with a set of parallel planes, however, is an ellisoid. It has been shown by BECKENBACH (1969) that the procedure mentioned causes an overestimation of LVV. If an ellipsoid of revolution is assumed for simplicity, and the angle between the long axis and the normal in the intersection point on the plane of the centerlines of the X-ray beams be α, the relative volume error is given by:

$$\varepsilon(\alpha) = \frac{V(\alpha) - V(0)}{V(0)} = \frac{1}{\cos\alpha} - 1 \quad \ldots \ldots \ldots \ldots \ldots \ldots (6.12)$$

This means that an error in volume of 10% is caused by false indication of the axis end-points with a divergence of $24\frac{1}{2}^{\circ}$; this holds regardless of the ellipsoid's excentricity.

So, it is obvious that for a correct calculation procedure the direction of the axis of the ventricle measured must be taken into account, as had been already indicated by ARVIDSSON (1961).

Furthermore, it has been shown from measurements on casts by WOOD (1972) that rotation around this axis causes an overestimation in the volume computed of up to 10%. A more refined model must therefore also account for the irregular shape of the left ventricular cavity, as a function of the angle of rotation, ψ.

The X-ray shadows represent this cavity including the *trabeculae carnae* and the papillary muscles. According to GRIBBE (1958,1960), their influence may amount to a gross : net volume ratio of 10:7, so a correc-

89

tion is necessary. For the papillary muscle a constant percentage of
14.5 is taken into account; the volume of the *trabeculae* is assumed to
vary linearly from 0% at end-diastole to 15.1% at end-systole.
This correction is included in the model proposed (VAN WIJK VAN
BRIEVINGH, 1973[a];1974[a]), which has been developed independently of a
view dependent correction-factor technique used in single-plane cineangiocardiography by SANTAMORE (1973).

So, improvement of the calculation of the LVV from biplane shadow
projections is expected to be possible when an anatomy-based model is
used for the calculation of LVV from these projections. This model has
to be constructed from measurement results obtained from casts and thus
gives a general indication for the shape of the LV. In order to be able
to use it, the human observer who draws the shadows with the light-pen
must provide extra information on:
1. the contraction phase of the heart at the frame under hand; this can
   be done on the basis of the ECG and LVP-curves as presented by the
   "Vidicor";
2. the direction of the axis in both projections, determining the angle
   of inclination α;
3. the value of ψ pertinent, to be estimated from the position of the
   heart relative to the projection system as judged from morphology.
   The line for $\psi = 0$ has been defined in the model at the middle of the
   intraventricular septum.
4. The type of heart under study, *e.g.* hypertrophic human, dog, pig, *etc.*
   for each of which a different set of values should be determined.

The geometric model has been constructed as follows. The casts, prepared
as described in the preceding section, were placed vertically on an optical bench, on which the X-ray source was represented by a light source
and the image intensifier by a transparent screen. Contours of the shadow
were drawn on paper for values of ψ from $0°-180°$ in steps of $30°$. There-
after, the casts were covered with transparent epoxy resin, and cut into
20 disks perpendicular to the axis. The shape of the LV-cast sections is
shown in Fig. 6.3, the + indicating the intersection with the LV-axis.

AORTA

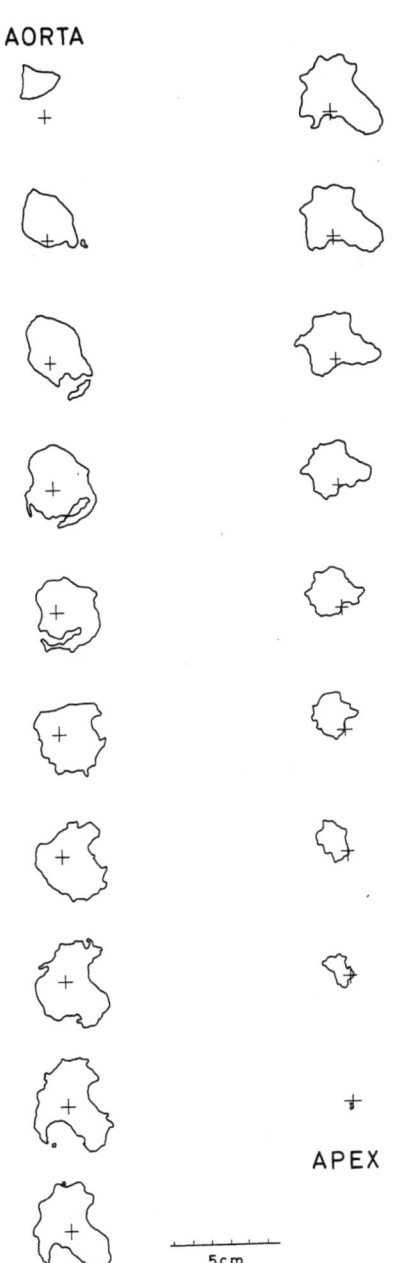

APEX

5 cm

Fig. 6.3 Shape of LV-cast Sections
    The numbering sequence of the slices is from the top
    to the bottom. (compare Fig. 6.4).
    It is clearly shown, that the shape of the slices
    cannot be closely approximated by ellises.

The area of the cast parts of the disks ΔA_i was determined by video-planimetry, corresponding perpendicular diameter pairs x_i', y_i' were measured from the shadow contours. The height, h, of the disks is given, so the volume of the LV may be derived from the partial volumes ΔV_i by

$$V = \sum_i \Delta V_i = h \sum_i \Delta A_i = h \sum_i f(x_i', y_i', \psi) \quad \ldots \ldots \ldots \ldots \quad (6.13)$$

in which formula the area of the slice is computed from the diameters x_i', y_i' for the given angle of rotation ψ.
A suitable expression for $\Delta A_i = f(x_i', y_i', \psi)$ is

$$\Delta A_i = \alpha_i(\psi) x_i' \, y_i' \quad \ldots \ldots \ldots \ldots \ldots \ldots \ldots \quad (6.14)$$

So, for each ith disk an "index of irregularity" $\alpha_i(\psi)$ has been computed, being the ratio of the area to the product of the perpendicular diameters corrected for projectional magnification, for each value of the angle ψ

$$\alpha_i(\psi) = \frac{\Delta A_i}{x_i' \, y_i'} \quad \ldots \ldots \ldots \ldots \ldots \ldots \ldots \ldots \quad (6.15)$$

The CHAPMAN, (1958) model assumes the slices to be elliptic cylinders, which means a degeneration of our model to $\alpha_i(\psi) = \frac{\pi}{4}$ for all i and ψ.
A set of casts, prepared from hearts arrested at known phases of contraction has been collected in order to compute values of α_i at various shapes of the ventricle. In Fig. 6.4 graphs of $\alpha_i(60^\circ)$ are given as an example of the ES- and ED- contraction state. The measurements have indicated that as the "impressions" into the casts made by the papillary muscles and the irregular surface have been accounted for, the dependence of α_i on ψ is not a very strong one.

After it had been shown that this model gave acceptable results in preliminary *in vivo* tests (VAN WIJK VAN BRIEVINGH, 1974[a]), the dependence on the angle of inclination α of the ventricle axis relative to the Z-axis of the coordinate system had to be established. The procedure as used by LANGE (1974) consists of fabricating several *replicae* of one cast

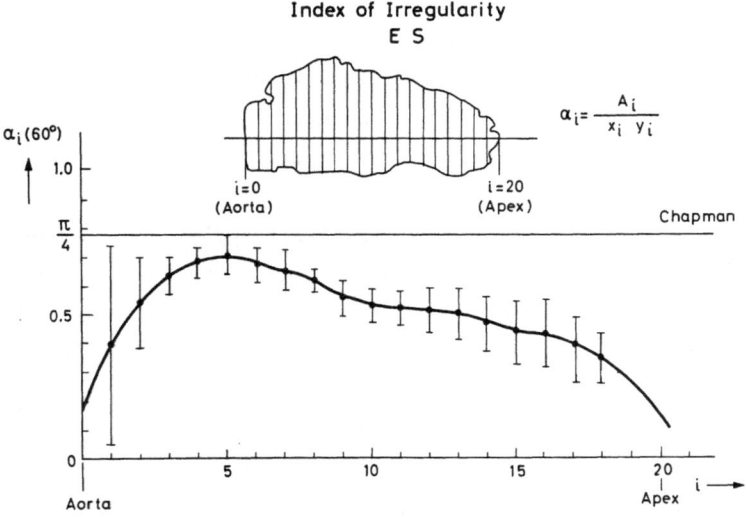

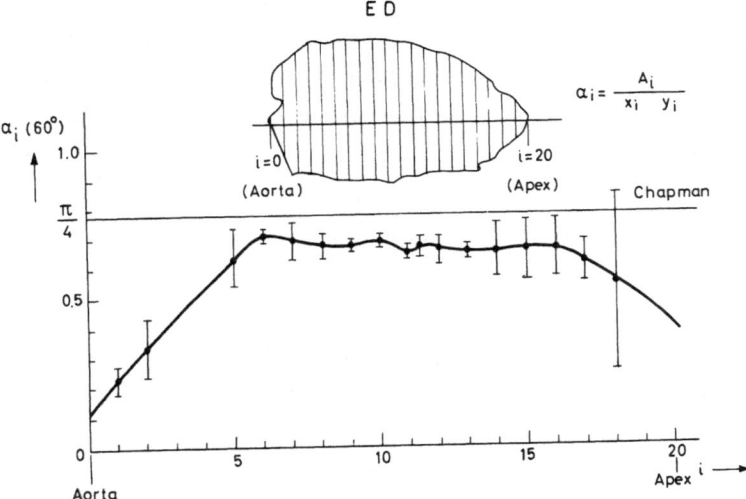

Fig. 6.4 Index of Irregularity
In this picture the shadow projections as well as
the "index of irregularity" curves are shown for
end-systolic (top) and end-diastolic (bottom) casts,
at a rotation around the ventricular axis of 60°.
Note that the curves lie below the constant value of
π/4. They represent mean values of ten ES and four
ED-casts, the vertical bars indicate the standard de-
viation.

by means of a mold of plaster, and cutting these mechanically with sets
of parallel planes under different angles. This is justified in the case
of casts of human hearts, which in general are very difficult to obtain.
As this seems a time-consuming procedure, however, if the model is to be
based on several ventricles instead of few, another approach has been
chosen by us. If not only the area but also the shape of the slices of
the LV-casts is taken into account, $e.g.$ sampled in polar coordinates
from the center (intersection point of the disk with the LV-axis) in
steps of six degrees by means of a digitizing table or by using the DCM
in combination with a TV-camera, a digitized description of the left-
ventricular shape can be given. On the basis of this description in
cylindrical coordinates a representation with a reasonable number of
parameters seemed possible. The reduction of the data was chosen in accordance with practical considerations (the number of slices) and the
interindividual variability within groups of hearts. We define a subspace M--the model chosen--of the multidimensional pattern space, in
which the shape of an LV-surface is represented as a point. Let a second
subspace S contain all points corresponding to ventricular shapes giving
the same biplane shadow projections. Then our model has to be chosen
such, that the disjunction between M and S is reduced to a point. Most
authors construct ellipses within the quadrilaterals formed by the tangent projection lines under various assumptions for the directions of
the ellipsoidal axes. Our model, based on the analysis of LV-casts, makes
use of a set of parameters describing the contours of the slices with
area ΔA_i, cut perpendicular to the main axis of the ventricle.
The technique of describing closed contours in terms of FOURIER coefficients is the same as will be mentioned in section VII.3. An example of
a synthesized and an individual slice contour enveloped by the same
quadrilateral, as well as an inscribed ellipse is given in Fig. 6.5.
A further reduction of the dimension of M was obtained by requiring
that the reconstructed contours which are bordered by the abovementioned
quadrilaterals have an area prescribed by the $\alpha_i(o)$, defined above. From
the set of parameters thus obtained, a "general" LV-cavity surface can
be constructed, fitting any pair of shadow projection contours of the

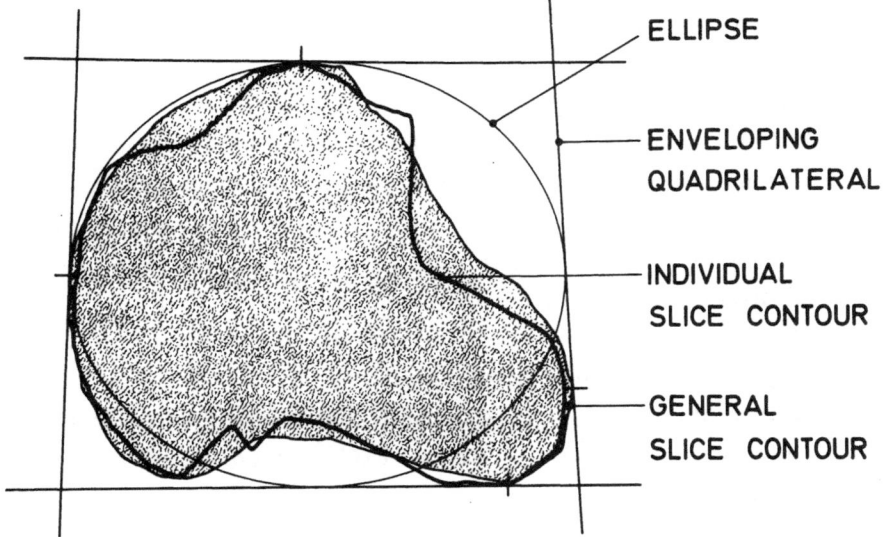

ELLIPSE

ENVELOPING
QUADRILATERAL

INDIVIDUAL
SLICE CONTOUR

GENERAL
SLICE CONTOUR

6.5 General LV-cast Section Contour
In this illustration the contour of a cast slice is shown, together
with its enveloping quadrilateral. The corresponding general contour
has been superimposed, showing the effect of the dispersion-weighted
transform. Apparently, this gives a better approximation than an el-
lipse would have yielded, irrespective of the orientation of its axes.

type of heart involved. As will be explained in detail in sections IX.3
and IX.4, the geometric enlargement factors and the orientation of the
ventricular axis as derived from its projections will be taken into account in this procedure (VAN WIJK VAN BRIEVINGH,1975).

95

5. *In Vitro Tests*

The accuracy of the correction procedure for projective enlargement,
of the calibration and of the geometric model have been established by
in vitro tests.

   a. Reconstruction of the true axis length in space.
A metal rod, bearing markers at a known distance has been placed in
various positions and under different known angles in the field of
view of the biplane installation. From their X-ray projections, as well
as dummy contours drawn with a light-pen, the programme described in
section IX.3 calculated the distance between the markers with an
error of 2.8%. (L_{true} = 33,5 mm; L_{mean} = 34.5 mm; s = 0.55; n = 10).

   b. Volume determination of a metal sphere.
As mentioned in section II.5, a steel sphere with a diameter of 75.00
mm has been placed in the field of view at different positions and its
projections recorded with various X-ray focus-image intensifier distances. The known volume was reproduced with an error of + 2.9% ± 2.5%;
the value calculated with the sphere positioned at the origin of the
X-ray beams differed as little as -0.04% from the true volume.

   c. Volume determination of LV-casts.
Casts of the left ventricle of the dogs sacrificed for the *in vivo* experiments described in section X.2 have been placed in the X-ray installation in various positions. The true volumes had been established
before, according to the water displacement method with an accuracy of
± 0.2%. Their shadow projections, available in hard contrast, have
been drawn with the light-pen, and their volumes calculated with the
geometric model described in the preceding section. A typical example
with V_{true} = 4.4 ml yielding a V_{angio} = 4.6 ± 0.2 ml (standard deviation
of 10 measurements).
This cast can be judged to represent the end-systolic case fairly well.

VII. DETECTION OF THE VENTRICULAR CONTOUR

1. Introduction

For several reasons, the X-ray shadows of the ventricle containing a
blood-contrast medium mixture are not fully relevant to the determination of its outline:

the mixing of the contrast medium with the blood directly after
injection is inhomogeneous;

in some pictures cavities containing the mixture and other structures overlap the left ventricle (LV);

the mitral valve is not clearly depicted when blood flows from the
left atrium into the left ventricle;

during the ejection phase, the aortic valve cannot be depicted, as
the ventricle and the aorta are both filled with the mixture;

at the location of the papillary muscles the concentration of
contrast medium is so small, that the "inner" part of the contour of
these muscles will be taken for the internal outline of the ventricular cavity if densitometric measurements are made.

Therefore, a priori knowledge on the LV-morphology has to be introduced
by a competent cardiologist, either in the on-line procedure or during
a preliminary and subsequent adjustment of densitometric equipment.

As already stated in section I.3, the design of the contour detection part of our system has been based on the considerations mentioned above. An attempt to describe quantitatively the influence of the experienced operator will be made in section 3 of this Chapter.

In literature, little is found about the ergonomic conditions under which the contours are drawn. The only aspect reported is the alternating viewing of moving short sequences of the cinefilm and still pictures (GREENE,1967; GRIBBE,1958), as small changes in LV-contour are more readily discernible if an image is remembered from the review. A modification of the video-disk control unit is under development, to achieve repeated presentation of tracks chosen for this purpose.

A method, which facilitates task division between the operator (pattern recognition and evaluation) and the computer (pattern manipulation and computation) makes use of an interactive display, but is limited as it is based on a particular (ellipsoidal) approximation for determining LVV (GOTT,1971; STIMSON,1972). The operator manipulates an elliptical cursor by software, displayed superimposed on the LV-image until he judges the fit to be best, after which LVV is calculated according to the ellipsoid model.

Several technical solutions of the contour determination problem are described. The carrier of the picture information may be cinefilm or a videosignal recorded on a magnetic medium; contour determination is found to be executed by hand or (semi-)automatically.

The oldest method for determining the LV-contours, still in use today, is drawing them on paper on which the cinefilms made during angiography are projected frame-by-frame as still pictures. This may be done with the help of front-surface mirrors to avoid distortion or loss of clarity (CHAPMAN,1958) onto a tracing platform, designed to receive slotting paper which can be fed into an optical scanner (BAKER,1961). The scanner converts the contours drawn with black ink into sets of diameters which are measured digitally and serve as computer input data. Other investigators use a special plotting projector with a transparant screen; the contours are followed manually with a recording coordinate system. The coordinates thus established are fed automatically into a tape puncher and then introduced to a computer (BJOERK,1970), or may be interfaced directly from a plotting table (BOVE,1970[b]; STEWART,1969).

If more simple geometric models are used to calculate the LVV, only axis lengths (GREEN,1967) or the main axis and area of the ventricle projections are used. Even if volume calculations are automated, a ruler and a mechanical planimeter are commonly used. (RACKLEY,1968; HAMNER,1969).

As more and more institutions felt the need of LVV-measurement, several technical solutions for digitizing contour data after manual tracing were developed. Analog-to-digital conversion of coordinates on a drawing board has been described (BRUN,1968,1970,1972), as well as a hand-held cursor transmitting coil in combination with a digitizing surface containing a grid of conductive strips (MILLETT,1971). The use of standard input devices as optical IBM scanner sheets for computer calculation is self-evident (GOERKE,1967).

Although digital handling of densitometric data offers many advantages, this approach has not been chosen for our investigation. In its recommendations on "Obtaining the maximum benefit of radiation exposure in diagnostic radiology through improved production and utilization of image formation" (1968), the NCRH Task Force on X-ray Image Analysis and System Design (section D, Machine Aided Feature Extraction) states:

> *1) The combination of a lightpen-like device, scanner and computer can provide great flexibility for quantitative measurement of radiographic images.*
> *2) The use of the image segment selector mechanism and computer appears to be a logical step on the road to complete automation of X-ray diagnosis."*

Automatic determination of the left-ventricular contour is considered impossible by some authors (CHAPMAN,1966).

During the discussion following the presentation of REITSMA's paper (HEUCK,1973, pp 134-136), HEINTZEN stated:

> *". . . möchte ich noch einmal vor der Illusion warnen, die Grenzen des linken Ventrikels vollautomatisch bestimmen zu können. An wirklichen Angiokardiogrammen musz dieses Verfahren so gut wie immer versagen, zu erheblichen Fehlbestimmungen führen oder eben nicht, wie oft vorgegeben, vollautomatisch sein . . . Auf Grund von örtlichen Dichtewerten und Dichtegradienten allein lassen sich die Kontouren des linken Ventrikels nicht festlegen. Eine grosse Zahl von dem Erfahrenen bekannten Formkriterien gehen in die Abgrenzung des linken Ventrikels mit ein."*

Volume determination based on automatic boundary detection in (cine-) angiocardiographs requires the solution of several problems, the first group of which has been mentioned in the beginning of this section. Secondly, the input of the densitometric picture data to the computer requires costly interfacing, in general using a flying spot scanner ETT,1971) or a programmable film reader (DESILETS,1971). The third group of problems is related to the algorithms used for boundary detection. Much theoretical work has been done in this field (ROSENFELD,1970). If a linear density profile may be assumed in the region where the boundary is expected, minimum variance and maximum likelihood methods may be used for contour determination (BECKENBACH,1969). Advantage can also be taken from the high degree of redundancy between successive images (KRUGER, 1971,1972,1973). A point of the contour may also be defined as the point of inflexion of a least-squares fitted 3rd degree polynomial (ROBB,1971), which may easily be computed.

A dynamic threshold method, which selects bimodal density histograms with large variances and estimates the composing distributions from them, appears to be a strong tool (CHOW,1970,1972). Digital processing of the image by logarithmic conversion, subtraction and averaging operations usually precedes the determination of histograms of regional density (CHOW,1971,1973). An algorithm for automatic detection of the aortic valve location has been described by GRIFFITH (1974).

2. *Semi-automatic Methods*

By its nature, an X-ray image intensifier - television system is extremely suitable for automatic densitometry as it incorporates fast scanning. If a plumbicon is used, it gives an electric output signal, with an amplitude which is in good approximation proportional to the local X-ray dose rate. Availability of fast analog-to-digital converters has led to the use of these systems as computer peripherals (DINN,1970; FROESCHLE, 1971; COVVEY,1971[a],1972). Direct use of such an interface for measurement of LV shape by densitometry has been reported (TRENHOLM,1972;1974). Properties of the currently available TV-systems with regard to spatial (BAILEY,1971) and temporal (FRANKEN,1972) resolution offer no severe limitations for use in combination with image intensifiers. Due to progress in the technology of the latter, however, use of special TV-systems instead of the usual types may be required in due time (see also section II.3.). Evidently, application of TV-techniques for several purposes in radiology and cardiology is abundant. To be mentioned here are the determination of heart wall motion during catheterization (LINDBERG,1972; MOND,1973; SCHMIEL,1973) and during recovery (LEVITSKY,1973); the automatic measurement of diameters (YIN,1972) and area (SIMON,1970; SCHELBERT, 1972; REITSMA,1973; MARCUS,1973) of the ventricular shadow. Furthermore, special instruments for LVV-measurement have been developed, which use (semi-)automatic analog contour detection from biplane roentgenographs (STURM,1968; RITMAN,1971; WOOD,1972; DAVIDSE,1974). The reconstruction of the irregularity formed ventricle from the contours so obtained poses principal problems (CHANG,1973) which limit the applicabillity.

In the systems mentioned above as well as in other "automated" methods (MARCUS,1972), the help of an operator is still required. In many cases, a monitor-lightpen combination is used for this purpose (HEINTZEN,1971[d], 1971[e]; ZIMMERMANN,1972,1973; ALDERMAN,1973). No references have been found, however, on the ergonomics involved in these systems nor on the influence of the a priori knowledge of the cardiologically trained observer.

3. *The Influence of the Trained Operator*

The contours drawn with the light-pen constitute the basis for the calculation of the left ventricular volume according to the geometric model
described in Chapter VI. The hypothesis to be proved is, that the density information in the pictures is not sufficient for the accurate determination of these contours, so that extra information on the morphology has to be introduced by a cardiologically trained human observer.
To do this, some characteristics of the man-machine part of the measurement system have been experimentally investigated. Especially the influence of a priori knowledge of the observer has been studied by comparing
the results of cardiologically trained observers with those of a group
having general medical knowledge only. The aspects of ventricular shape
(frontal and lateral projections at end-diastolic and end-systolic
moments) and the concentration level of contrast medium have thereby
been taken into account. To this end, firstly the conditions under which
the observer has to draw the contours with a light-pen on a television
monitor screen had to be optimized according to ergonomic principles
(WHITHAM,1964), resulting in the design of a special console shown in
Fig. 7.1, (VULKER,1975; internal report) and in the prescription of the
ambient illumination (McCORMICK,1970; VAN MEETEREN,1973). The properties
of the TV-monitor play an important role,in this respect and have been
taken into account[']. In order to make the investigation possible it is
necessary first to provide a quantitative basis for the comparison of
the human operators behaviour. It has to be examined whether the hypothesis that a cardiologically trained observer makes use of his a priori
knowledge of the cardiac structures in his judgement of the X-ray picture is correct. If so, the contours and axes drawn by this observer
provide a better basis for the LVV-calculation than those drawn by a
naive observer. As the accuracy of the volume measurement is among
other factors determined by the geometric model

[']Personal Communication of A. Franken, Medical Systems Division,
Philips, Eindhoven (1973).

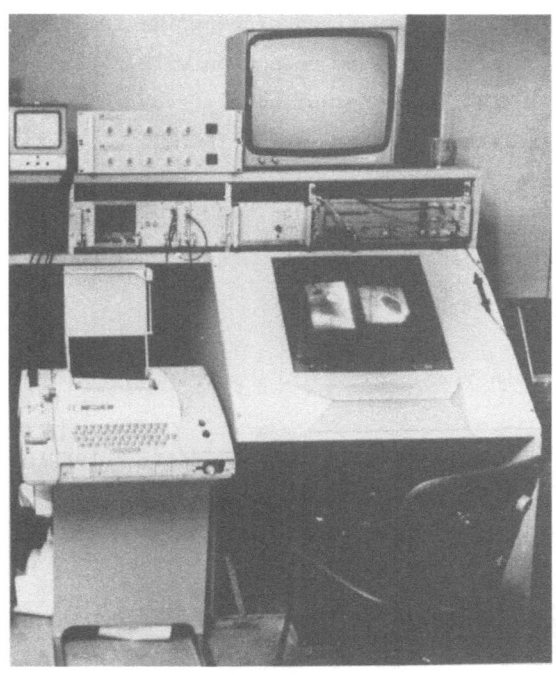

Fig. 7.1 Console for Contour Determination
In the rack on top of the console and the teletype
are placed (from left to right): Anacor output part,
serial input buffer and digital contour memory.

used to calculate the LV-volume from contour- and axis direction data, this investigation is restricted to the two quantities last mentioned. The ventricular axis direction in space can be derived from its orthogonal projections. Calculation of the least-squares best fit of a straight line from manually drawn axes poses no problem, and comparison can be based on the parameters of the analytical representation of the lines. For the comparison of the contours drawn, however, a different criterion has to be chosen. To this respect, distinction should be made between the variations induced by hand motorics for the general shape of LV-shadows and the procedure of judgement applied to contour determination. The criterion may be a different one in both cases. In redrawing a contour presented with sufficient contrast and resolution, local deviations are of prime importance, whereas in the second case these cannot be separated from judgement errors.

No general theory for the comparison of experimental curves is available (BLUM,1964); the criteria have to be chosen with regard to the special problem at hand. In the judgement of consistency in redrawing contours, no direction of preference can be given. Therefore, a criterion based on the area enclosed by the contours drawn may be the most relevant one. To account for variations with both signs, the area difference alone is not sufficient, and an absolute value measure must be used. A simple way to accomplish this, is to take

$$(A \vee B - A \wedge B)/(A \vee B). \quad \ldots \ldots \ldots \ldots \ldots \ldots \ldots \ldots \quad (7.1)$$

if A and B are the closed curves to be compared, interpreted as region boundaries in a VENN-diagram (Fig. 7.2)

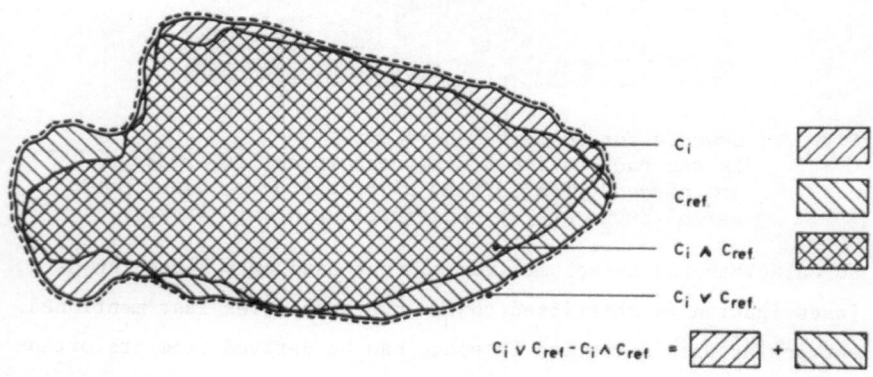

Fig. 7.2 Area Criterion for Comparison of Contours

This procedure seems suitable because the reference curve is predetermined. In the second case, the contours are drawn from one and the same X-ray picture, but it is not possible to define this in terms of density gradients, because of the very nature of the problem posed.

Thus the curves obtained from a group of cardiologically trained observers and those drawn by a control group of naive operators have to be separated. In this approach, the "mean curve" of the first group is the most appropriate basis for comparison, so an *ad-hoc* definition of this quantity must be given. As the contour coordinates are found relative to a set of axes determined by the position of the X-ray sources and image intensifiers as described in section II.4, they are dependent upon the location of the subject under the biplane installation and thus fairly arbitrary. Reference points in the anatomical structure are difficult to give and are in general inconsistent because of respiration and cardiac contraction movements. So, a reference has to be found relative to the ventricular contours themselves.

A description of the shape of biological structures with a set of parameters is required in many cases, *e.g.* for cells in microphotographs of muscle preparations (VENEMA,1974) or for the reconstruction of the placenta position from ultrasonic reflection patterns. Electric field distribution calculations within the torso require data on the contour of transversal slices of the body (BARNARD,1967) as does the computation of radiation treatment plans in radiotherapy (CLARKE,1969). For closed curves as of interest here, description in polar coordinates seems indicated, as long as the resulting function is defined unambiguously. It is evident that this method is sensitive to the position of the origin relative to the contour. As a first step, the center of gravity of the curve has been chosen for the origin, and the zero argument direction in parallel to one of the axes in the original orthogonal system. So modulus *vs.* argument graphs can be constructed for experimentally found contours, as shown in Fig. 7.3. The corresponding functions are of a periodic nature and satisfy the DIRICHLET conditions, so Harmonic Analysis may be applied. This procedure then supplies a way of making a better estimate for the origin: if a maximum fraction of the total "signal energy" is contained in the lowest order term of the FOURIER series expansion, the origin position is considered optimal['] .

['] Personal communication of A. van Oosterom, Laboratory for Medical Physics, Municipal University of Amsterdam.

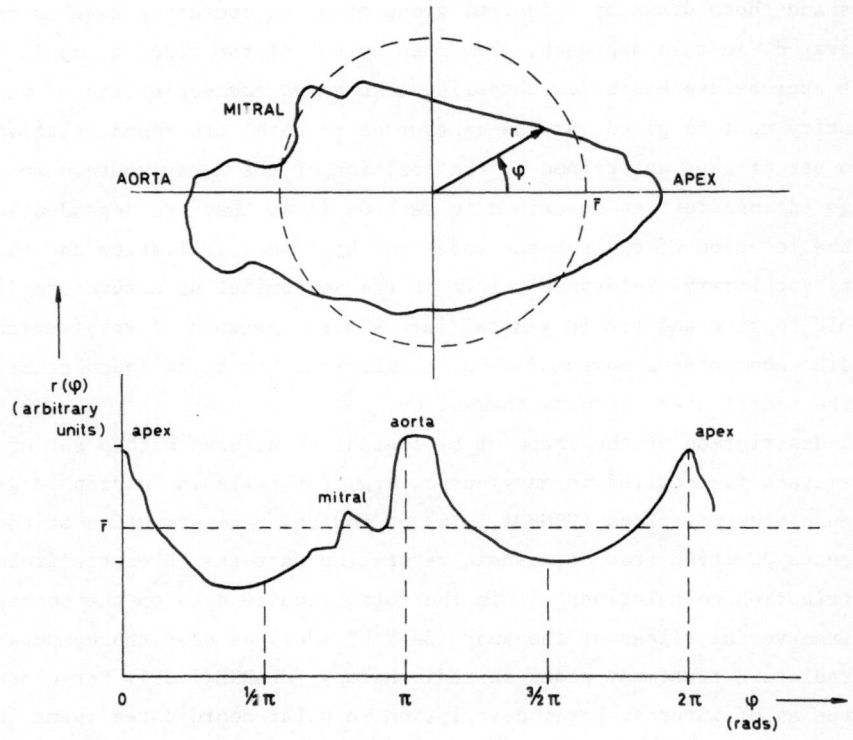

Fig. 7.3 Polar Representation of LV-contour

Then the contour can be described by the coefficients c_n in a TSCHEBYCHEFF polynomial expansion of the function $f(x)$

$$f(x) \simeq \sum_{n=0}^{m} c_n T_n(x) \quad . \quad . \quad . \quad . \quad . \quad . \quad . \quad . \quad . \quad . \quad . \quad . \quad . \quad . \quad (7.2^a)$$

$$c_o = \frac{1}{\pi} \int_{-1}^{+1} \frac{f(x)}{\sqrt{1 - x^2}} \, dx \quad . \quad . \quad . \quad . \quad . \quad . \quad . \quad . \quad . \quad . \quad (7.2^b)$$

$$c_n = \frac{2}{\pi} \int_{-1}^{+1} \frac{f(x) T_n(x)}{\sqrt{1 - x^2}} \, dx \quad . \quad . \quad . \quad . \quad . \quad . \quad . \quad . \quad . \quad (7.2^c)$$

$$T_o(x) = 1; \; T_1(x) = x; \; \text{and} \; T_{n+1}(x) = 2x T_n(x) - T_{n-1}(x) \quad . \quad . \quad . \quad (7.2^d)$$

with the $T_n(x)$ the TSCHEBYCHEFF polynomials of the first kind.
This series converges more rapidly than the expansion in any other set
of orthogonal polynomials does, the error being limited in its absolute
value rather than in its root-mean-square value. The c_n are defined
by the integration operation, which is linear, so they are applicable
to the calculation of the mean and of the variance between several
curves by performing the proper calculations on equally-numbered coefficients. Segments of interest selected in the curve to be analyzed
may be transformed linearly to the $(-1,+1)$ interval. This means, that
after the whole contour has been analyzed, *e.g.* with regard to the
inter- or intra-individual variability, the parts exhibiting the largest
variation may be studied seperately. The procedure will be described
in more detail in section IX.6.

Parameterization of curves is a key problem in pattern recognition
(FREEMAN, 1961). A method, using FOURIER descriptors for plane closed
curves, which gives results that are invariant to scale, translation
and rotation, has been described by ZAHN (1972). Therefore, it is
applicable to an analysis of the shape of the contours drawn by the
human operators, but cannot serve for reconstructing a "mean curve"
according to location and size. Values for the mean and variance of
equally-numbered sine and cosine coefficients, however, can be exploited for comparison purposes. It should be noted that this would
not hold for a FOURIER expansion in terms of amplitude and phase,
because of the non-linear operations by which these are derived from
the sine and cosine coefficients. ZAHN (1972) also has presented a
reconstruction theorem for contours from their descriptors, which is to
be used for visual comparison of the synthesized curves.

According to the principles mentioned, the influence of the human
operator as a "black box in a white coat" can be analyzed with respect
to:

hand motorics, including tremor, by the "relative absolute" error
made in redrawing a predetermined curve in high contrast;

correct judgement of the left-ventricular contours from a set
of angiograms in different projections, contraction phases, and

with different levels of contrast medium concentration, in terms of coordinates;

correct judgement of the corresponding long axis projections, corresponding with the same set of pictures;

the shape of the contours drawn, without regard to size and position.

These aspects can be described quantitatively by the parameters discussed above. So, the influence of the operators' a priori knowledge can be determined from these data by Analysis of Variance (SCHEFFE,1959). The shape description method is also used in determining the "general slice contour" of ventricular cast slices as mentioned in section VI.4.

4. Conclusions

The simplest method for comparing contours which should have been drawn identically, is the "unity minus intersection" criterion, mentioned in the preceding section. An average set of contours (A) has been redrawn by 7 observers, a random example of which (B) is also depicted in Fig. 7.4.

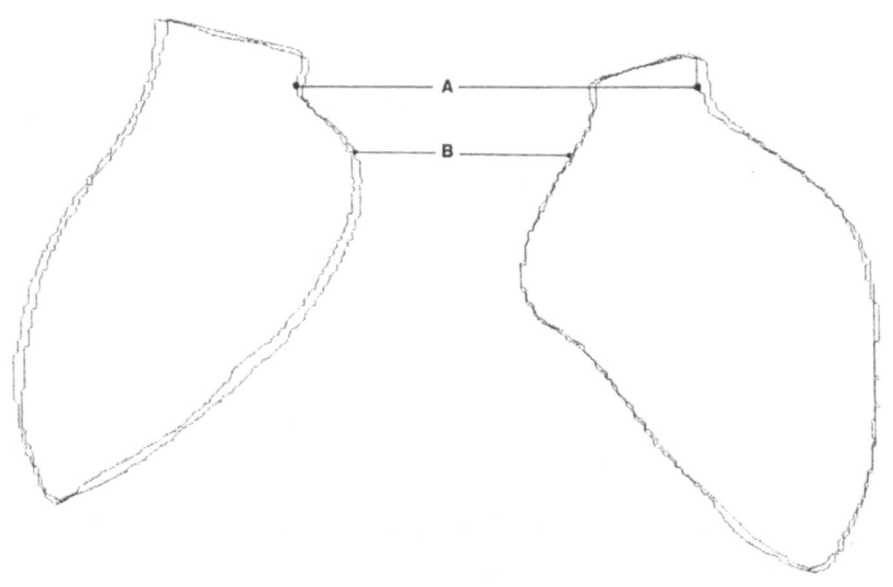

Fig. 7.4 Example of Area Criterion

The criterion gave a result of 1.6% ± 0.5, indicating that the operator together with the subsystem light-pen-monitor-DCM is limited only to a small extent by hand motorics and discretization.

In order to obtain an impression of the sensitivity of the shape description methods, the contour shown above has also been submitted to the corresponding analysis. The spectrum of FOURIER coefficients according to ZAHN (1972) has been plotted for the whole contour, whereas the set of coefficients in the TSCHEBYCHEFF expansion has been calculated for the apical region ($\phi_1 = \pi/4$; $\phi_2 = -\pi/4$), see Fig. 7.5.

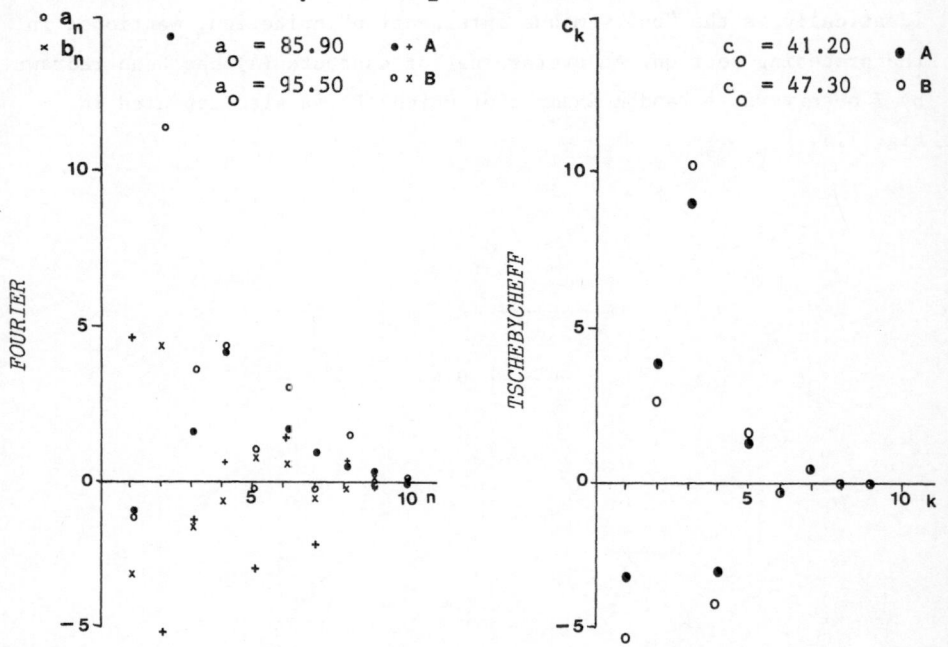

Fig. 7.5 Example of Shape Description

From these spectra it appears that about 16 and 5 coefficients respectively are sufficient for an adequate description in the two cases.

The results of a preliminary investigation according to the method described have been used for estimating the uncertainty intervals in the process of drawing contours and axes (see section XI.2). During the experiment it became clear that the operators did not have a sufficiently consistent interpretation to make a statistical evaluation meaningful.

It is concluded that the human observer has to be trained in drawing contours and axes with respect to the model used, in order to obtain the full benefit of the method.

VIII. DATA CONVERSION

1. Introduction

As discussed in the preceding chapters, the data gathered become available in various forms. In order to apply the calculations necessary for
the determination of LVV and derived quantities, as well as for a presentation which is useful to the clinician, processing of these data is
required. To this end, hardware and software procedures have to be applied in an efficient combination. After the preprocessed pictural information has been presented to the human operator under optimal ergonomical circumstances, the contours and axes drawn are to be entered into
the computer together with other measurement data and system parameters.
In this process, identification and time relationships must be retained.
Corresponding data have to be labelled in such a way that organizing
them in files in the computer's memory becomes possible. Furthermore,
the judgement and drawing procedures performed by the human operator
are time consuming, the price to be paid for an improvement in accuracy.
Under these circumstances, the evaluation procedure should be kept as
simple as possible.

In the following sections, the light-pen system to be used by the
operator will be described. The contour and axis data are retained in a

digital contour memory, into which the "Anacor" data of the corresponding frame are inserted automatically. All other relevant data, as introduced into the "Digicor" previously, are read-out automatically via a second interface. Special sorting programs take care of the organization of the data in a predetermined file structure.

2. Light-pen System and Contour Memory

As described in section VII, a trained operator draws the contours of both LV-projections with a light-pen while selected individual TV-frames are presented as still pictures from the videodisc. In doing so, he bases himself on the information contained in the monitor picture as well as on his a priori knowledge of the anatomical structures. The contour coordinates are retained in a digital contour memory (DCM). During the evaluation phase, also the ten TV-lines containing "Anacor" information are coupled to the DCM by means of a line selector/videoswitch. By this procedure, the contour as well as the corresponding analog data are entered. Thus the time relationship between physiological signal values and X-ray picture data are preserved. The light-pen/contour memory system as a part of the data transfer hardware is depicted in Fig. 8.1.

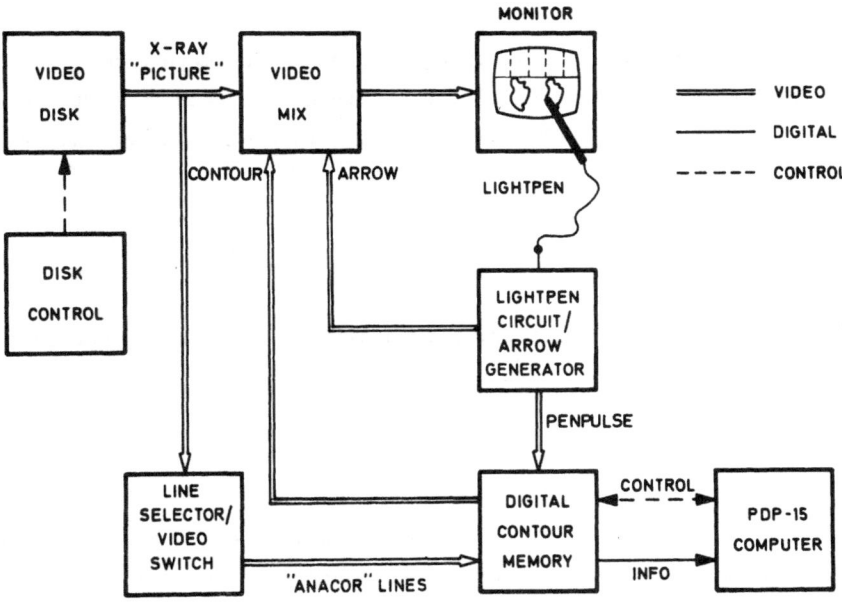

Fig. 8.1 Block-diagram of Data Transfer

113

As a television monitor is in principle a temporal-to-spatial converter, a light-pen producing an electric signal upon each passage of the electron beam, which may be put in temporal relation to the scanning pulse pattern, is a suitable means to determine the coordinates of the point indicated on the screen (PILZ,1964). In roentgenographic pictures, the average screen brightness is low, so a sensitive photo-electric device is required. To ensure a reliable functioning, many systems produce a light-emitting area in the vicinity of the point indicated, *e.g.* a cross (ALDERMAN,1973), a retangle (ZIMMERMANN,1973) or even the bright, blank raster of a second monitor (COVVEY,1971[b]; HEINTZEN,1973). Unlike the light-pens used in graphical computer displays, no software search for the pen position is necessary, and the use of replayed video frames eliminates flicker problems regardless of the number of points displayed. From an ergonomical point of view, a light-pen is to be preferred to a joy-stick (WISCOMB,1971) or to a set of cross-hairs manipulated with a pantograph (HEINTZEN,1973).

The light-pen systems mentioned above require an image memory to record the contours drawn. The bistable screen of a scan converter or a track of a videodisc (SOUTHWORTH,1968) are in use as analog memory elements.

The light-pen system used in our installation consists of the following parts, as shown in the block-diagram of Fig. 8.2.

Monitor-light-pen combination, with amplifier and arrow generator;
Digital contour memory, with controlcircuit;
Position counters, with switched oscillator;
Interface, inclusive parallel input buffer.

This system is an improvement over those described elsewhere since the spatial resolution limitations of the scan converter used previously have been overcome, and the light-pen function is independent of the local brightness of the monitor picture. The light-emitting arrow generated is composed of parts of eight TV-lines which are given higher brightness, and may be chosen in an arrow-like pattern based on ergonomical considerations.

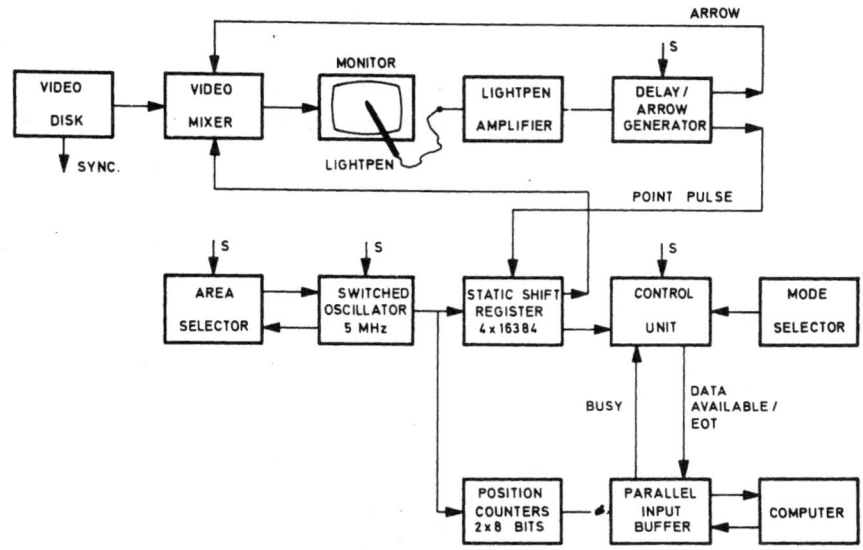

Fig. 8.2 Light-pen System

The upper left-hand corner of the periphrased rectangle of this arrow corresponds with the point recorded in the contour memory. The light-pen consists of a light-sensitive diode[1] used in such a part of its characteristic that a compromise between sensitivity and noise is found. A preamplifier stage incorporated in the pen-holder also gives the necessary low output impedance. At each passage of the electron beam in the monitor, a pulse is generated, the instance of occurence of which is related to the scanning pattern by counting line synchronization and

---

[1] Monsanto MD 2.

clock pulses. The contents of the position counters give the coordinates of the point indicated by the light-pen. The output of a static shift register, clocked synchronously with the synchronization pulse pattern has been coupled to the input. Each time a light-pen pulse is generated, a "1" is introduced into the corresponding section. At the command of the register output, the videosignal is switched to the "white" level during 200 ns after a delay of one frame, if a "1" occurs. Thus the line drawn by the light-pen is made visible on the monitor. If a pedal is pressed, a "0" is put into the register section corresponding to the image point indicated by the pen; in this manner parts of the contour may be erased. An example of an LV-contour drawn is given in Fig. 8.3.

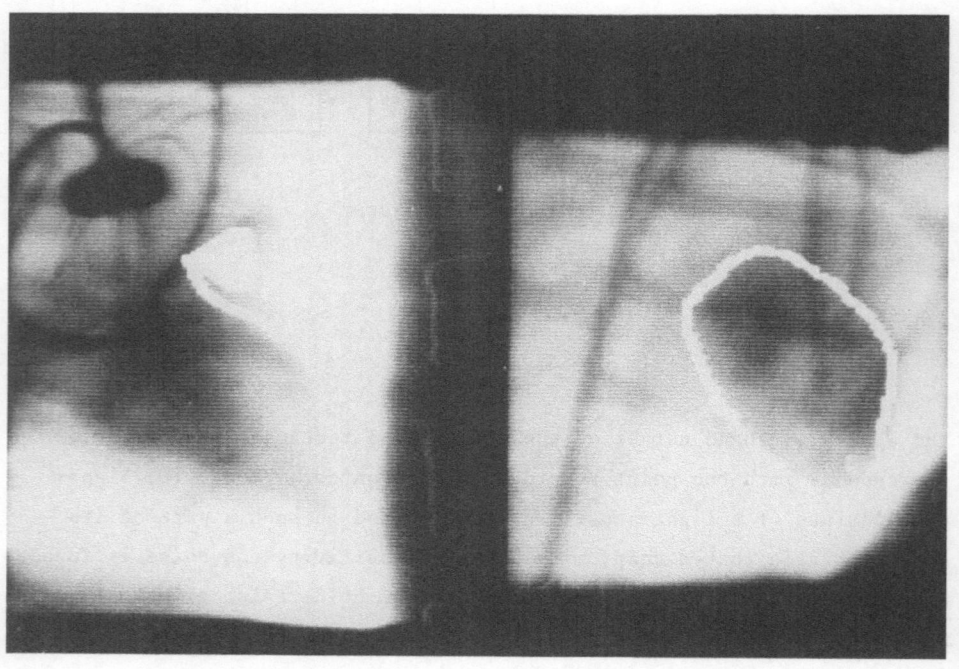

Fig. 8.3 Example of LV-contour

The availability of fast static shift registers made the use of digital contour memories feasible (VAN VEEN, internal report M 107); this solution has the additional feature that interfacing to a computer may be easily performed. The higher price, compared with dynamic shift registers, is compensated by the obviation of intricate control circuits and the possibility to read out the memory either in the video mode or at the command of the computer with the help of a standard teletype interface, which facilitates data handling considerably. Great practical advantages in comparison with the scan converter used previously are that the removal of parts of the contour drawn is easily achieved and that the spatial resolution is about twice as good. The DCM has a working area of 256 image points over 256 television frame lines, chosen with a line selector switch. As the spatial resolution should be equal in horizontal and vertical direction, each image point has a duration of 200 ns. Thus, a resolution of about 1 mm on the screen of a monitor with a 20" screen diagonal is reached. The static shift register has to accomodate $(256)^2 = 65536$ bits, which are retained in 64 units of 1024 bits [1], organized in four decks because of the maximum clock frequency of the register elements. Each point is characterised by three quantities:

y-coordinate, found by counting line synchronization pulses.
x-coordinate, found by counting 5 MHz clockpulses.
z-coordinate, the memory content, being "1" for the contour and "0" for all other points.

To use the DCM as a computer peripheral, its output has been made compatible with the computer teletype receiver [2] which requires eleven bit words consisting of one start bit ("1"), eight data bits, and two stop bits ("0") respectively. At the command of a 100 kHz clockpulse oscillator, the x and y coordinates, containing eight bits each, of only those points of which the z-coordinate has the logical value "1" are read-out consecutively into the input buffer register and sent to the computer upon a "data available"/"non-busy" combination. As soon as the last point of the array has been reached, the control is given back to the 5 MHz clock so that the DCM works in the TV-mode again. As an indication of this condition, the z-coordinate of this lower right-hand point is also sent to the computer, regardless of its logical value.

(The system in its final form has been developed by A. Richtering Blenken)

---

[1] SIGNETICS, type 2533
[2] DEC, type M706

3. *Digicor*

The Digicor output section behaves like a computer peripheral of the pseudo-teletype kind. Its memory may be coupled to a teletype transmitter, which at the command of the interface sends its data words as fast as the computer can accept them. A block-diagram of the output situation is shown in Fig. 8.4.

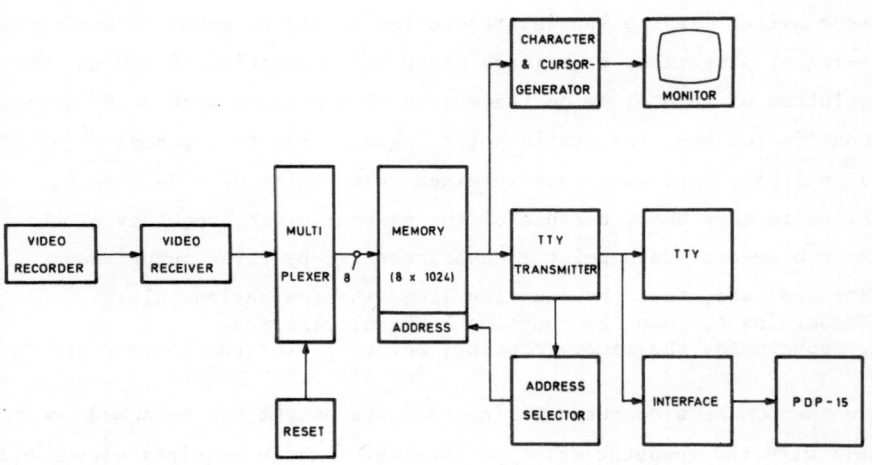

Fig. 8.4 Digicor Output Section

If the computer read-out mode is chosen, the videosignal from the videodisc, containing a "still picture" selected, is fed to the video receiver. The lines containing digital information are selected, the signal is decoded, checked on parity and converted into 7-bits words.
All words detected from the message inscribed in the first set of 25 lines of the frame are entered into the memory. Words in which a parity-failure had been detected are marked with an extra bit. From the recording of the message in the second set of 25 lines, only those words are entered which have such a marked memory address as their destination.

Thus, faults which have occured in the first set of lines can be corrected from the repeating of the message. Should a word be marked as faulty in both messages, the extra bit gives an indication of this situation. On the monitor screen, the corresponding alphanumeric character is then underlined for this purpose. After input into the computer, this condition may be selected by software. In a second read-out mode, to be chosen with a switching circuit, the transmitter is coupled to a teletype, to produce a hard copy of the recorded message for filing purposes if required.

4. *Evaluation Procedure*

As already mentioned in the introduction to this Chapter, efficiency of
the evaluation procedure is an important factor. Dependent on the aspects
relevant to the diagnosis of the patient, a selection of pictures to be
submitted to quantitative elaboration has to be made. In section V.5.
the possibilities of archivation have already been discussed, which are
necessary as the videodisk acts as an intermediate memory only. In this
phase, the medical doctor responsible for the patient must take part.
The detection of the contours and axes in the pictures chosen, however,
may be the task of a medical technician specialized in this field. The
procedure to be executed is depicted in Fig. 8.5., which is largely self-
explanatory. In step 8, a verification possibility has been included,
in which the contours and axes drawn are presented superimposed to the
operator in the form the computer will evaluate them, when desired after
a preprocessing in which interpolation of missing points and exclusion
of parts of a contour inadvertently drawn with more than two points per
television line. The circle phantom picture is available in maximal contrast so that it can be introduced via the same level discriminator as
the calibration values of "Anacor" data. The contour of the sphere phantom shadows, however, have to be drawn by hand. The calibration program
in which the phantom data are exploited has been described in section
II.5. A special-purpose terminal including a microcomputer for executing
the evaluation procedure upon push-button command is under investigation.

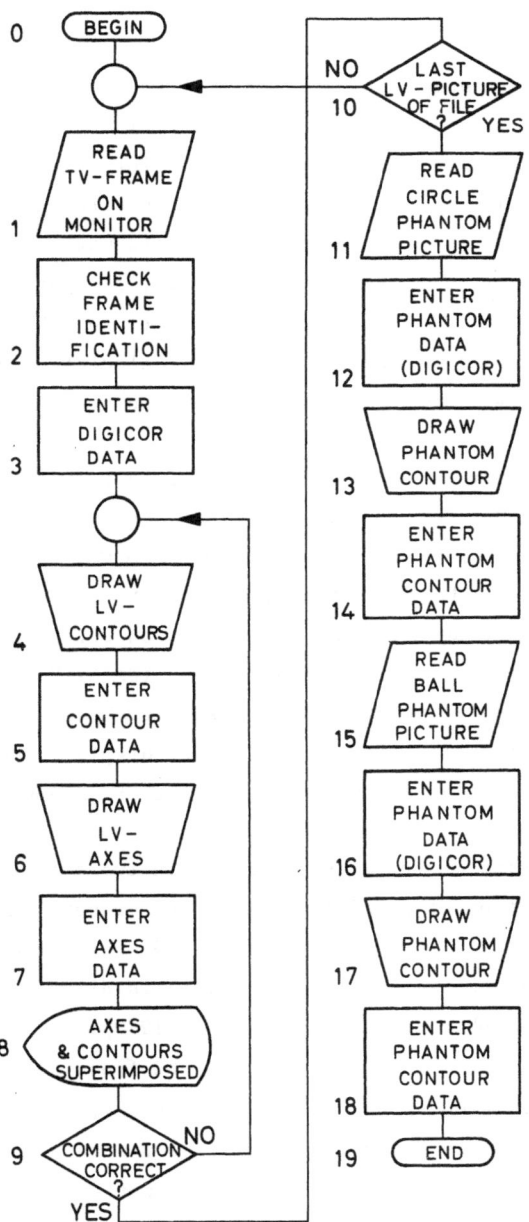

0   BEGIN

10   NO   LAST LV – PICTURE OF FILE ?   YES

1   READ TV-FRAME ON MONITOR

11   READ CIRCLE PHANTOM PICTURE

2   CHECK FRAME IDENTI-FICATION

12   ENTER PHANTOM DATA (DIGICOR)

3   ENTER DIGICOR DATA

13   DRAW PHANTOM CONTOUR

4   DRAW LV – CONTOURS

14   ENTER PHANTOM CONTOUR DATA

5   ENTER CONTOUR DATA

15   READ BALL PHANTOM PICTURE

6   DRAW LV – AXES

16   ENTER PHANTOM DATA (DIGICOR)

7   ENTER AXES DATA

17   DRAW PHANTOM CONTOUR

8   AXES & CONTOURS SUPERIMPOSED

18   ENTER PHANTOM CONTOUR DATA

9   COMBINATION CORRECT ?   NO   YES

19   END

Fig. 8.5 Flow-Diagram of Evaluation Procedure

5. Data Presentation

After introduction of the basic data into the computer as described in
the preceding section, the geometric model is to be applied, whereby the
projective enlargement factors are taken into account. Since patient
data and measurement parameters as well as calculated values are recorded in one file, the presentation of results may be chosen in relation to
the requirements of clinical use. Firstly, all patient data should be
put on paper by a line printer in a format, suitable for filing with
the patient's status. On this document, calculated values, *e.g.* cardiac
output, average values of ejection fraction, EF = SV/EDV, and stroke
work SW = $\oint$ pdV, *etc.* are also recorded. These values are made comparable
with other patients' data by normalizing on the basis of the body surface area (BSA), yielding cardiac index, volume index, *etc.* Then, data
calculated on a beat-to-beat basis are presented in tabulated form on a
second sheet. In the third place, sampled data of LVV, pressures, and
other measured quantities can be plotted as curves *vs.* time; smoothed
according to proper numerical procedures (DA SILVA,1974, internal report
M 116). Representative graphs of these curves and of the PV-diagram may
be chosen by the clinician on the visual display, and then added to the
patient's file in hard copy from the plotter. Examples are given in Fig.
8.6.

The recording of ventricular images in two orthogonal planes allows
the determination of spatial location and measurement of change in position of the heart. Besides the analysis of wall movement, the creation
of a three-dimensional contraction model is also feasible by means
of computer graphic techniques (SANDLER,1970). The model may be displayed from different viewing aspects and frame rates. Since the
heart has been reconstructed within a cartesian coordinate system,
spatial movement is directly determinable. Groups of dots are displayed
in a triangular or rectangular geometric pattern, thus giving a visual
description of the ventricle's surface. By relating the pattern to a
reference direction (*e.g.* to a light source assumed to shine on the
image) a shading is included. The programme has to suppress those

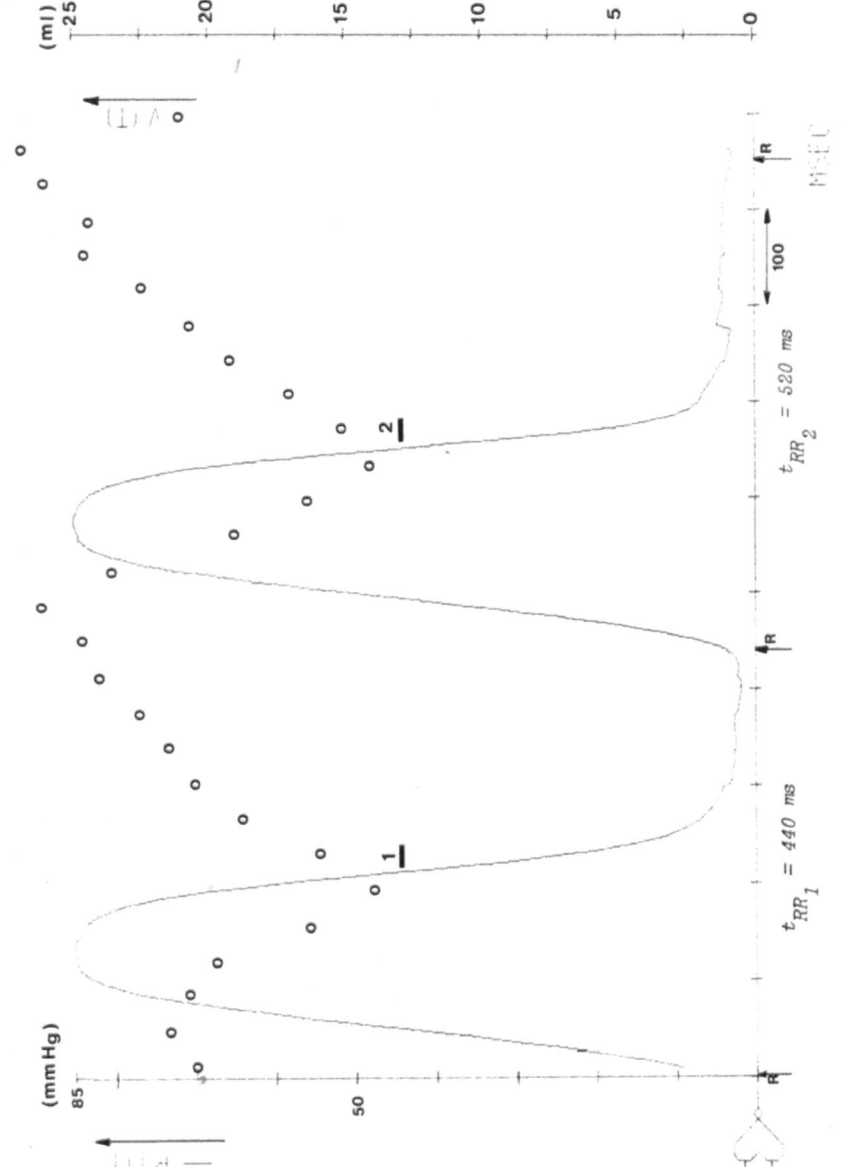

Fig. 8.6^a LV- Pressure and Volume vs. Time

123

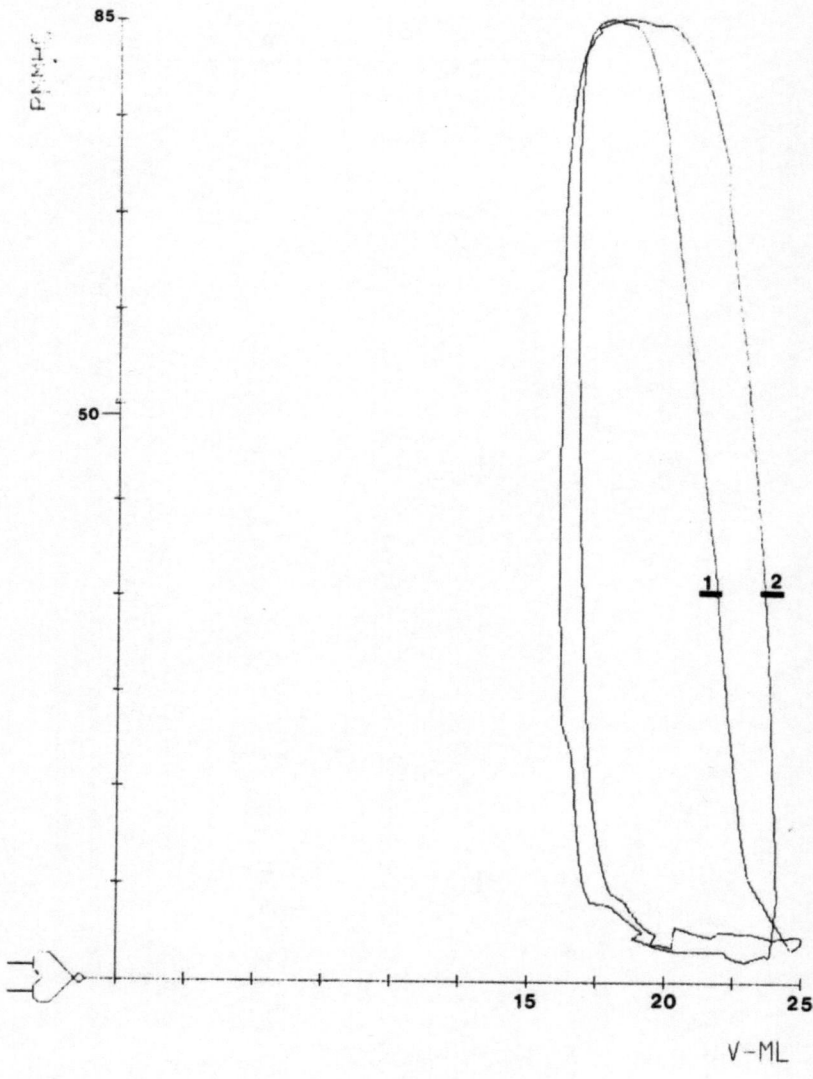

Fig. 8.6^b Pressure-Volume Diagram

parts of the surface which are "hidden" at the time of display. The display routine also may rotate the data into the desired viewing position, and create a perspective view (COULAM, 1972). By means of the videodisk a sequence of images as displayed on the scan-converter in a time-lapse mode by the computer for successive instants of time may be recorded and played back with a desired time-base. As all information other than the margins of the left ventricle is eliminated by the procedures described, the viewer is able to concentrate solely on the dynamic motion of the ventricle. The LV-shape displayed is dependent on the geometric model assumed, the movement pattern on the frame of reference. Most authors use the anterioposterior and lateral diameters of the ventricular shadow projection contours as main axes of ellipses, which are stacked to form the whole surface image. In our programme a general shape of slices perpendicular to the ventricular axis is assumed, as explained in section VI.4. Two types of pseudo-threedimensional presentation of LV-shape are used by us. The first one gives a picture on a TV-monitor from a scan-converter memory screen. In this case, a modified z-modulation may be used to yield a more suggestive picture. Besides, the presentation is generated within a few seconds and thus may be chosen in interaction with the operator until a satisfactory view is obtained. The programme is based on the already mentioned publication of COULAM (1972). The second one bears a close relationship to the model used in volume calculation. It is used for documenting in plotted form the shape of a ventricular cavity. The left-ventricular shape is of a complexity precluding a detailed computation of its dimensions from only two orthogonal projections, but the a priori information introduced by the model makes a general impression feasible, as shown in Fig. 8.7.

In the choice of the data presentation, the user should be guided by a programmed interaction scheme, which also performs checks on the data asked for (RECOURT, 1972). The evaluation of this programme is carried out in close collaboration with the medical staff.

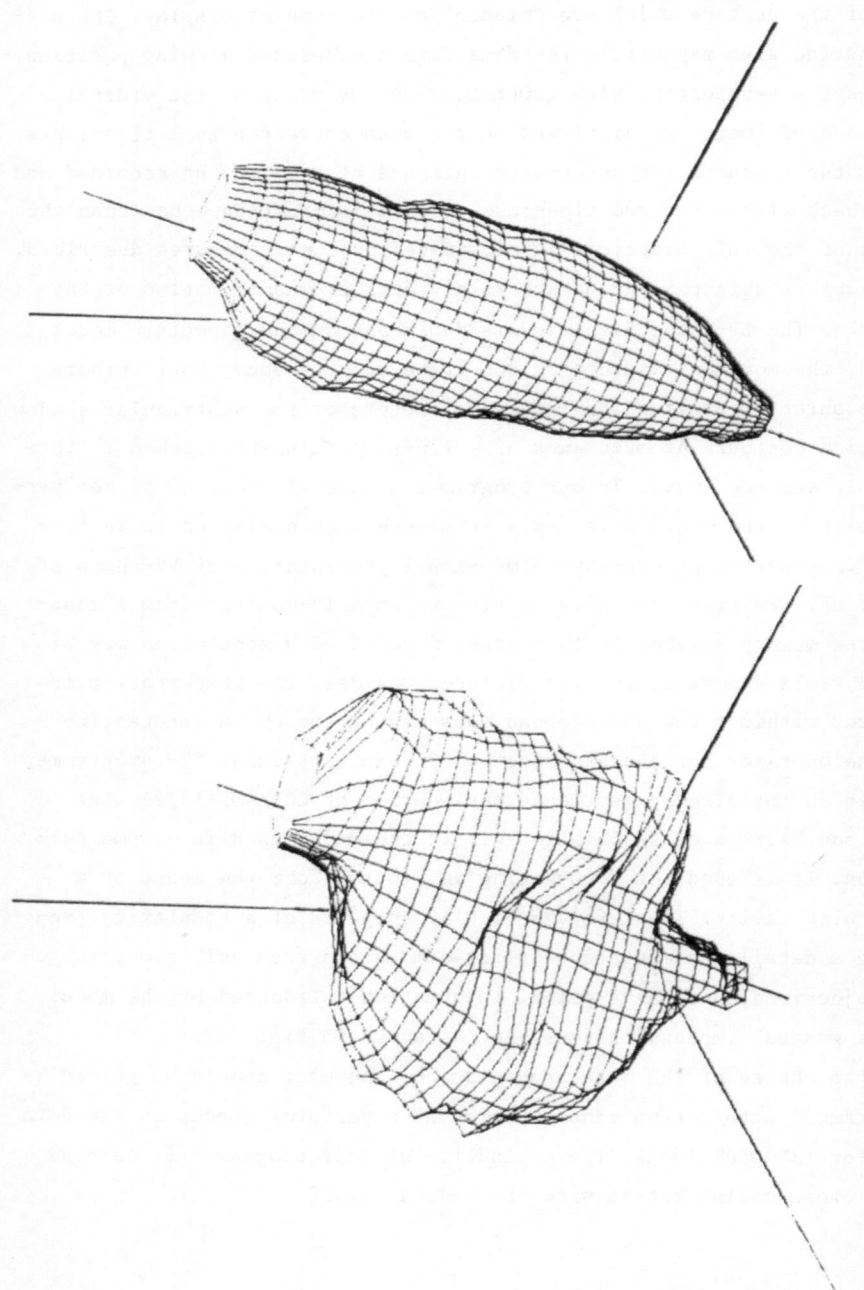

Fig. 8.7 Example of pseudo-3D Hard-copy Output
Left: End-diastolic.
Right: End-systolic.

IX. THE SOFTWARE SYSTEM

1. *Introduction*

The calculation of LVV from the contour- and other data, as well as the
computation of derived quantities (stroke work from PV-relation, ejection fraction, regurgitation fraction, correlation with other parameters
e.g. RR-intervals) has to be performed with a digital computer. As mini-
computers are becoming less expensive every day, the use of these may
be considered if a self-contained LVV-measurement system is to be developed. The programming has to be done in machine code in this case.
If computing facilities are already present, either from a central in-
stitute or in the clinic, limitations in core memory space may be present. In general then, a monitor programme services various users on a
time-sharing basis. Under these circumstances, a modular structure of
the software package is of importance.

The data acquisition and processing as described in the following
paragraphs, is performed by means of a medium scale computer (DIGITAL
EQUIPMENT PDP-15) of the Dataprocessing Centre of the Utrecht Department of Cardiology (CGC). The system is depicted in Fig. 9.1. This computer system possesses, besides many standard peripherals *e.g.* tape and
disk units, several special purpose peripherals, which are, among others,

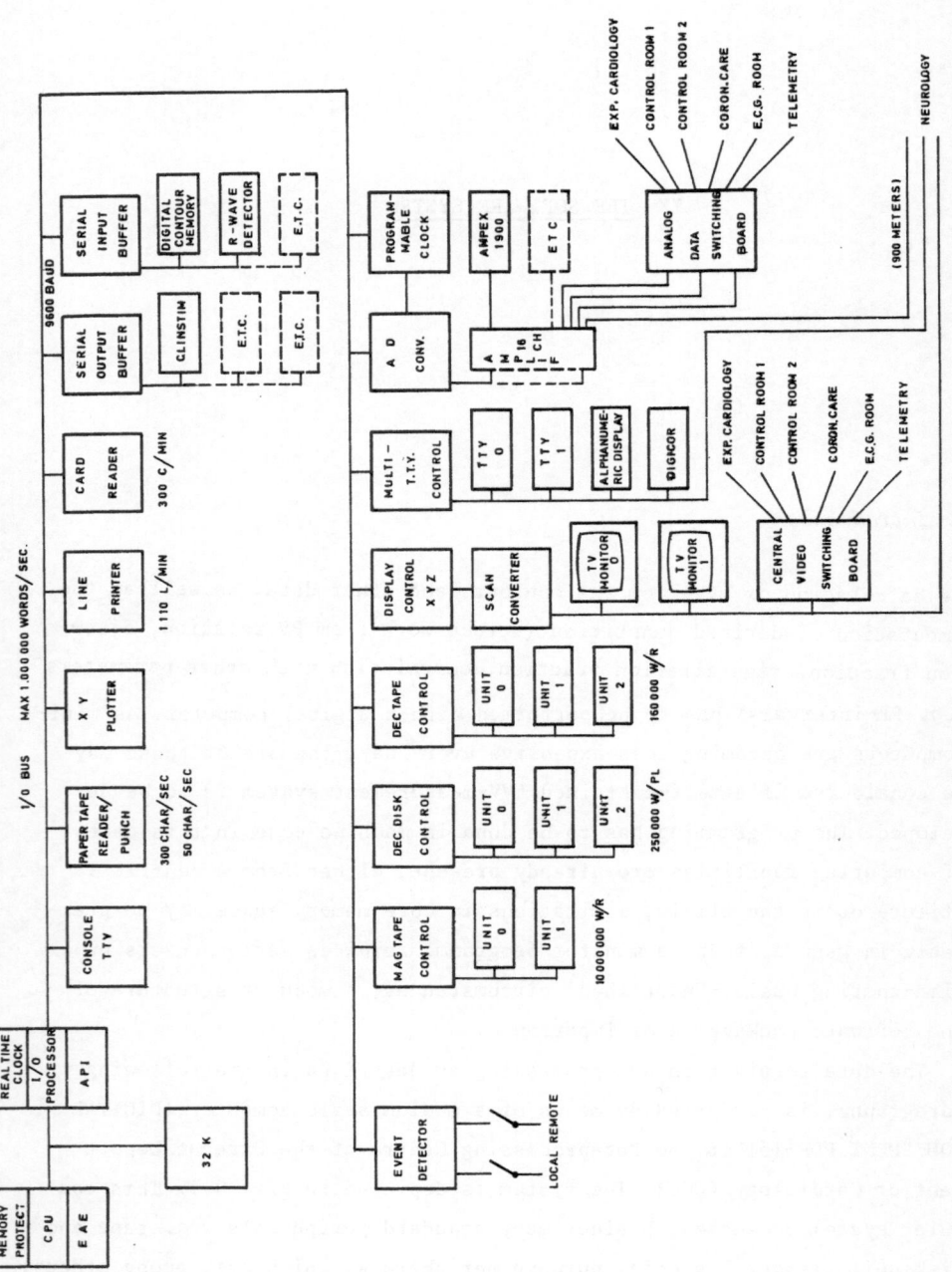

CENTRAL COMPUTER GROUP CARDIOLOGY, UNIVERSITY OF UTRECHT

128

used for the LVV-project (scan converters, clinical stimulator, digital contour memory). The laboratories of the department are connected with the computer by means of video-, analog-, and digital switching stations. The computer is running under a multiprogramming system (RSX), which grants the possibility to service more than one user at a time.

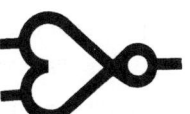

More detailed information on the software package as described in this chapter may be obtained from the Data Processing Centre of the Department of Cardiology, Academic Hospital of Utrecht, 101 Catharijnesingel, Utrecht, The Netherlands.

2. Modular Structure

An operating system as described above implies that a user can have the disposal of only a small part of the core memory. At the moment this part is fixed on 4 k words; when the core memory is expanded to 48 k, this will be 12 k words. The construction of extensive overlay structures is indicated under this operating system, if larger programs have to be executed. The software package for the acquisition and processing of data related to the LVV-project is of a modular structure, containing one module per function performed. This has the advantage that new functions may be simply added, and that modules to be changed or deleted may be excluded without affecting the structure itself. As shown in Fig. 9.2., a manual input device, mostly a video display unit or a teletype, is used to control the programs via a "MAIN" module which is the only part of the programme which stays resident in the core memory. Dependent on the operator's instructions, one of the other modules is called into this core memory from disk; during the use of the system each module overlays its predecessor, thus saving memory space. The loading of the modules is performed by the "CONTROL" module; intermediate results of calculations are retained on units of the "DEC-tape" or "MAG-tape" type.

The "INPUT" module performs the data acquisition. Data from the Digicor (patient information *etc.*) and data from the DCM are read into the computer memory and written in tape structure "A". If the data on tape A contain information on phantoms, the "FANTO" module is used to process this information. For testing the software package without the Digicor and the Digital Contour Memory connected, a "PAPER" and a "PAPIN" module have been added. These modules produce and process respectively a papertape, punched according to the contour memory and Digicor formats. Information from the left ventricle itself is processed by the "VOLUM" module, which produces a tape structure B. From this tape B, several types of output may be chosen, *e.g.* a table from the line printer, pseudo-threedimensional presentations on the scan converter screen or plotter, and pressure or volume *vs.* time curves. To this end, a "DOCUM"

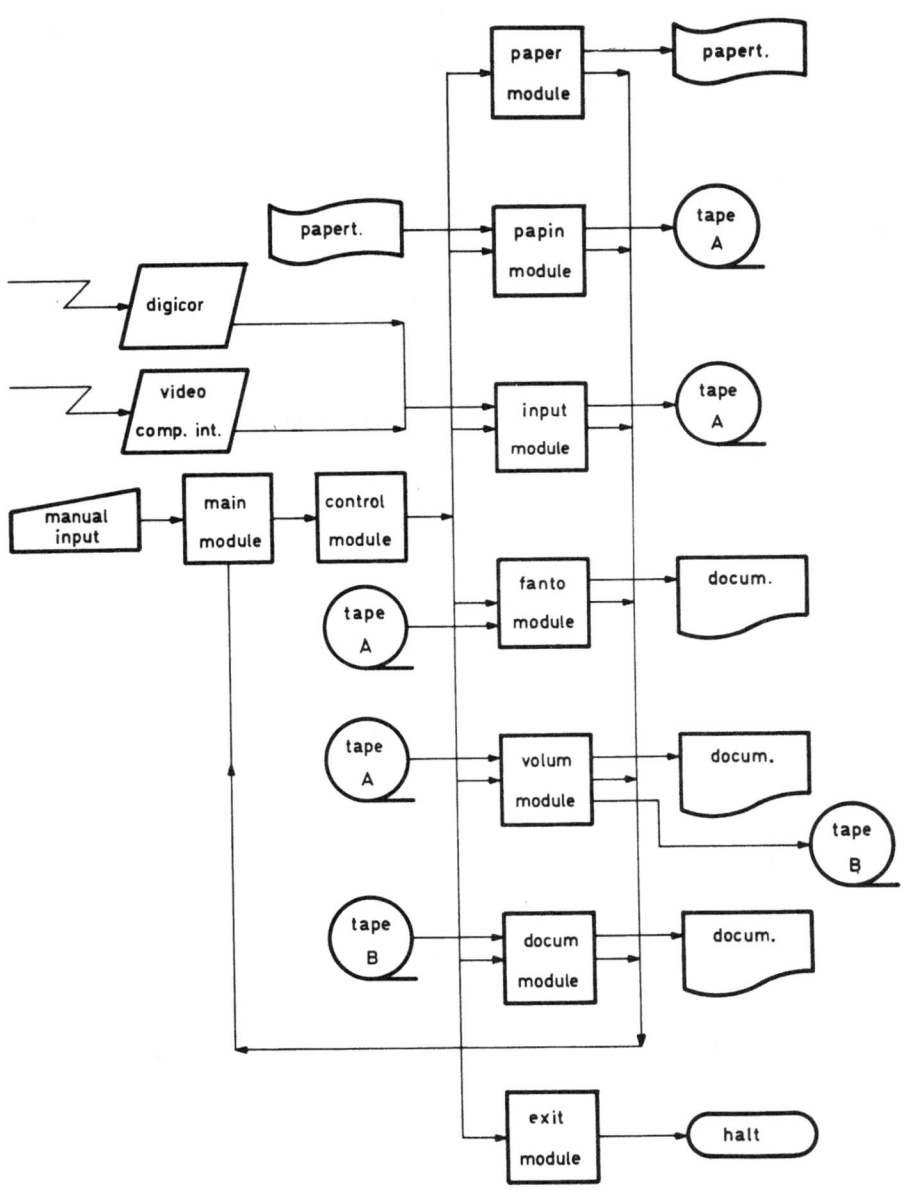

Fig. 9.2 Modular Structure of Software Package

module has been added. This program includes the use of a smoothing sub-routine, (DA SILVA,internal report M 116), which applies a procedure based on spline functions as described by REINSCH (1967). This has been proven necessary, as the sampling frequencies of 25 Hz (fields) and 50 Hz (frames) are low, and points are unevenly spread along the PV-curve. A correlation "CORRE" module will be added to the system, in order to establish the relationship between the quantities measured and the duration of preceding RR-intervals, as discussed in section I.1.

The run is closed if the module "EXIT" is called, and control is returned to the "MAIN" program again. This set-up results in a flexible and relatively simple use of the computer by the operator and an effective use of its capacity. It has been developed under the creative supervision of R. van Poelgeest.

3. Data Conversion

As mentioned in the preceding section, the data corresponding to selected parts of the measurement are divided into files. The volume module
and related subroutines are loaded upon a call statement, in which also
has to be specified whether a new calibration must be used. If so, first
the circular phantom data are read-in, from which the least-squares best-
fit circles in the two projections are computed, the centres of which
will be used as origins. From the known radii the calibration factors
in both planes are determined as described in section II.5. Furthermore,
the calibration of the "Anacor" channels is determined from this calibration frame in which known input voltages are represented by the distances between pulses, converted into counter units.

Next, frame pairs containing corresponding ventricular axis- and contour data are read-in. Two straight lines are least-squares fitted to the
axis points and the equations of the same are calculated, as well as
the spatial direction of the ventricular axis, expressed by the angles
β and γ (Fig. 9.3). The contour data are interpolated so that a closed
curve is obtained, as the subroutine for the determination of the con-
tour-axis intersection points cannot handle curves with missing points.
As mentioned in section VIII.4, the interpolated contours and the fitted
axis projections may be presented to the observer for final approval by
means of the scan-converter graphical display. From the intersection
points and the axis position, the end points and true length in space of
the ventricle axis are determined. This procedure does not necessarily
yield a unique result. In practice, it has been shown that the lower
endpoint of the axis, L_2, (corresponding to the ventricle apex) is determined uniquely, whereas for the upper endpoints, L_1, different values
may be found from both projections. If the distance between the two
upper points on the axis is greater than 5% of the axis length
($L = \overline{L_1 L_2}$), a mean value is used and the resulting volume marked during
output. After this, the ventricle axis in space is divided equidistantly
into n-1 sections ($h = L/n-1$), with n equal to the maximum number of
contour point pairs (the number of TV-lines containing contour data)

in the projections.

As shown in Fig. 9.3., in all intersection points, P_i, planes A_i are erected through the X-ray tube foci, F_1 and F_2, (hatched). The intersection lines of these planes with the XOZ and YOZ-planes are a_i and b_i respectively, subtending angles α_{1_i} and α_{2_i} with the X and Y axis directions. These lines naturally pass through the shadow projections P_i' and P_i'' of the intersection point P_i on the projections $L_1' L_2'$ and $L_1'' L_2''$ of the ventricle axis $L_1 L_2$. The lengths of the intersection segments of a_i and b_i with the ventricular shadow contours C' and C'' constitute the "contour diameters" x_i and y_i, respectively. From these, the "equivalent diameter" pairs x_i' and y_i' have to be determined in order to apply the volume model. This procedure, as illustrated in the insert of Fig. 9.3., includes the magnification factor correction. The end-points of x_i and y_i are connected with F_2 and F_1, respectively; the connection lines intersect $F_1 P_i''$ and $F_2 P_i'$ at the end-points of x_i' and y_i'. It is clear that x_i' and y_i' do not coincide with the "true diameters" connecting the tangent points of the ventricular surface with the X-ray beams as used by BESSE (1974). Instead, the equivalent diameters and indices of irregularity constitute the basis of the volume calculation procedure proposed. This is justified by the sensitivity of the calculation on the direction of the true diameters, which may change considerably due to small irregularities on the LV-surface.

4. Volume Calculation

From the data, converted as described in the preceding section, the left ventricular volume may be calculated according to various models. In order to be able to obtain results comparable with those reported in literature, the area-length model (DODGE,1960; NELSON,1966) and the ellipsoidal slice model (CHAPMAN,1958) have been programmed also. The first one utilizes the main axis end-points for determination of the long axis of an ellipsoid, the minor axes of which are calculated from the areas enclosed by the contours in both projections. The second one assumes the diameters of the contours to be the axes of elliptical cylinders which together make up the total volume. For both models, regression formulae based on comparisons with casts, have been calculated (BENTIVOGLIO,1972; HEINTZEN,1974), and taken into account by us.

Our model, as explained in section VI.4, makes use of "indices of irregularity" which are used as multiplicative constants to calculate from each set of diameters--computed as described in the preceding section--the area of general cylinders of known height (the distance along the ventricle axis between intersection points). The volumes of these are added according to SIMPSON's rule. As the irregularities in shape are already included in the model, no regression formulae will be required (VAN WIJK VAN BRIEVINGH,1975). Having available the set $\{x_i',y_i'\}$, the array $\alpha_i(\beta,\gamma,\psi)$ corresponding with the type of heart and contraction phase has to be applied. This is performed by calculation of the areas $\Delta A_i(\beta,\gamma,\psi)$ of the ith slice of the ventricle model in the same orientation, positioned correspondingly. Hereby, the general slice shape as described in section VI.4. is used. Observations on casts have shown that for the various models the indices of irregularity $\alpha_i(\beta,\gamma,\psi) = \Delta A_i/x_i'y_i'$ deviate little from their mean values, so that they may be used as a good estimate for the situation *in vivo*.

The calculation procedure as performed in steps by the computer is shown in the "volume" module's flow diagram of Fig. 9.4., details are explained in the caption.

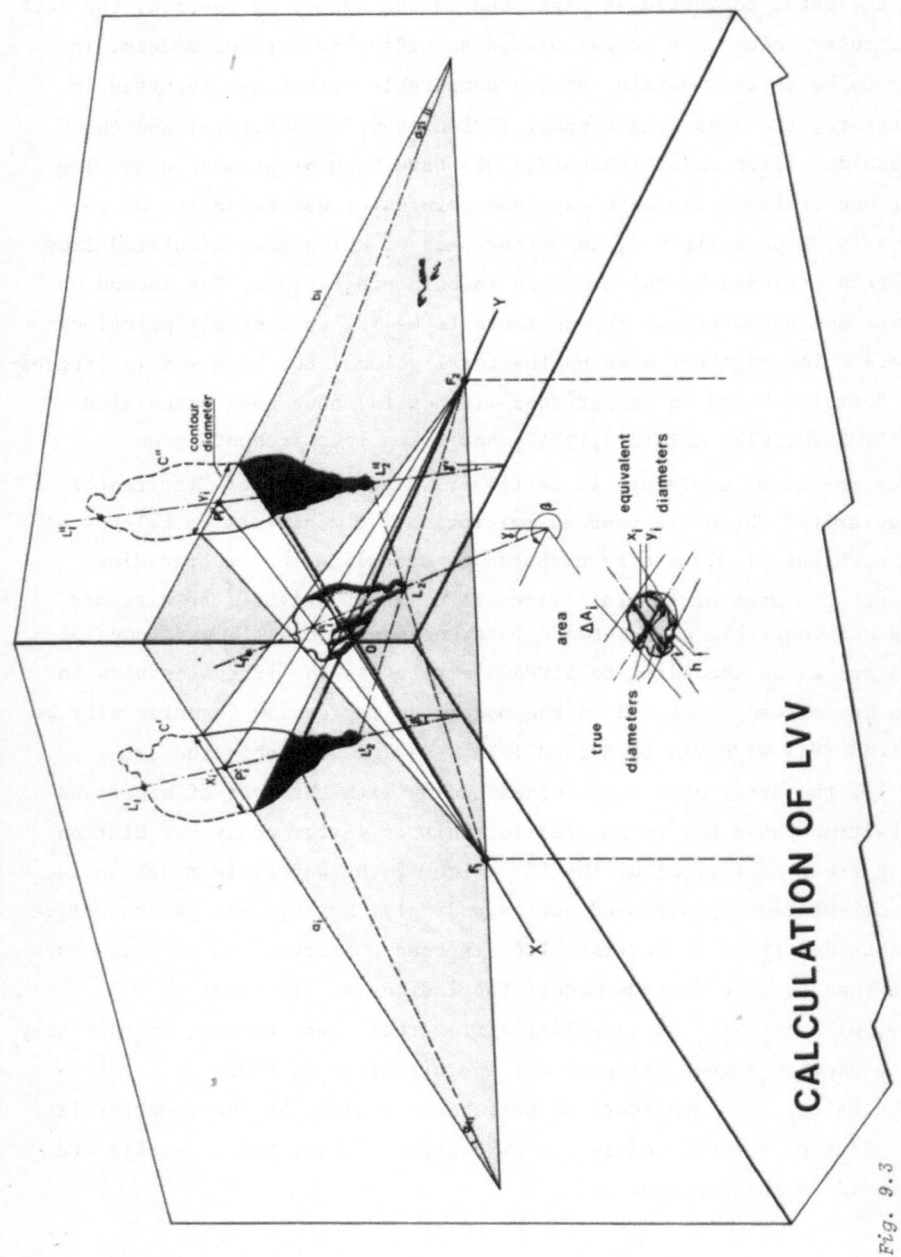

CALCULATION OF LVV

Fig. 9.3

In this flow-diagram two "judgement loops" are shown.

The determination of the intersection points of corresponding contours and axes in both projection planes is crucial to the correct calculation of the ventricular axis position in space. Therefore, the combinations of the reconstructed contours with their least-squares best-fitted axes are presented for visual inspection first. After possible correction also the end-points found can be presented on the scan-converter visual display.

These facilities may not be used in the evaluation of each frame, but have proven useful in doubtful cases. They will also be used for instruction purposes.

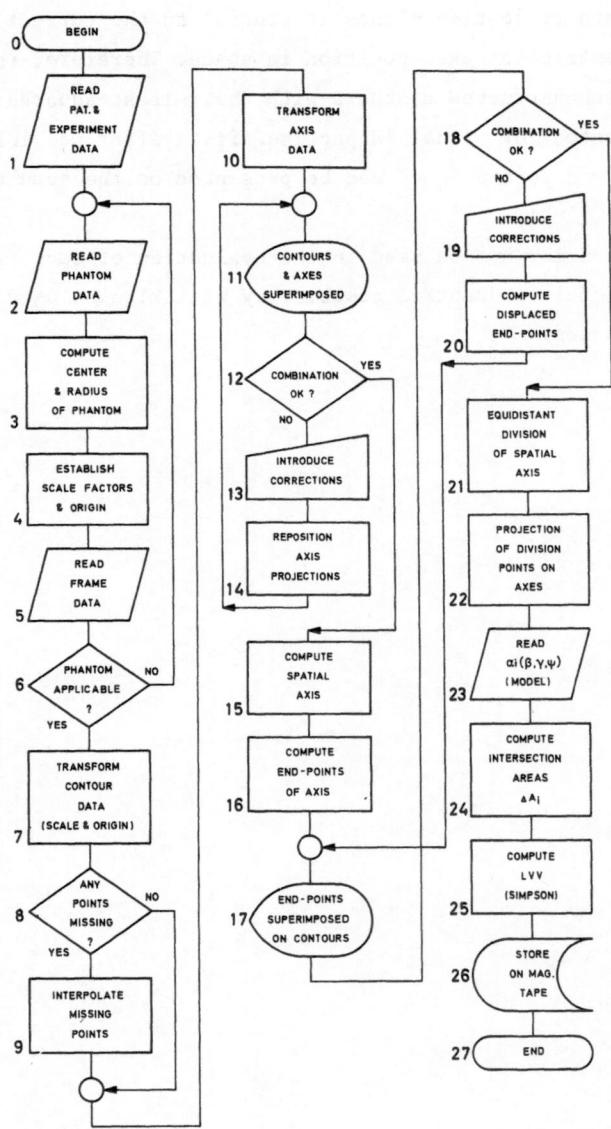

Fig. 9.4 Flow-diagram of "VOLUM" Module

Fig. 9.4   Flow-diagram of "VOLUM" module

0. The "VOLUM" module is loaded by the "CONTROL" module.
1. Identification data and system parameters (*e.g.* the distance of the X-ray foci and image intensifier entrance windows relative to the intersection point of the main axes) are read from MAG tape A.
2. Contours drawn from the circular slit phantoms are read from tape A.
3. The centers of gravity of these contour points are computed; from the distance to these centers the radii of the least-square best fitting circles are determined.
4. From the coordinates of the centers and the known radii of the circular slits, scale conversion factors are computed.
5. Sets of data (LV-axis and contour projections), are read from tape A.
6. These sets bear a reference to the phantom data; if the reference is changed, steps 2 through 6 are repeated.
7. The contour data are transformed according to the conversion factors sub 4 and thus expressed in mm with reference to carthesian systems with the centers computed sub 3 as origins.
8/9. Missing or superfluous points are filled in or eliminated respectively, by a selective recognition from groups of neighbouring points.
10. Transformation of the axis data as described sub 7.
11/14. Corresponding sets of contours and axes are displayed on a TV-screen by means of a Scan-Converter acting as an output peripheral. Thus the relative position of axes and contours may be checked. If repositioning of the axes is required, this may be performed at the command of teletype.
15. From the axis projections in both planes, the spatial direction of the ventricular axis is computed.
16. The end-points of this axis in space are computed from the intersections of the axis projections with the contours.
17/20. As the results of (16) are crucial to the following calculations, another visual judgement procedure with correction capability is introduced.
21. The LV-axis in space is equidistantly divided into a number of sections about equal to the number of TV-lines of the smallest contour.
22. The intersection points are projected back to the axis projections to give an equal number of non-equidistant points there.
23. According to the angles β and γ of the axis inclination computed and the rotation angle ψ given, the relevant geometric model array is called. From this array the "indices of irregularity" for the contraction phase at hand as introduced previously are taken.
24. With the α_i, the elementary slice areas, ΔA_i, are computed from the corresponding diameter pairs, according to the "general slice shape".
25. From these areas and the thickness of the slices, h, the total left ventricular volume, LVV, is calculated according to SIMPSON's rule.
26. The results are stored on MAG-tape B, which is to contain all primary and calculated data for each frame.
27. The control is rendered to the "MAIN" module if all frames of the file have been handled.

(Programmed by J. Heethaar).

5. *Data Presentation*

For the presentation of results and other data as described in section
VIII.5, many routines for hard-copy output and for visualization on a
display exist. Some of the special procedures essential to our system
are briefly described here.

5.1. Smoothing_procedure

The blocks of data, organized in the file structure on tape "B" refer to
various moments with respect to the cardiac cycle. A special "Anacor"
channel gives the time, elapsed since the preceding R-wave of the electrocardiogram. The sets of samples corresponding with individual heartbeats
may be selected from these time intervals, and form the basis of the
smoothing procedure (DA SILVA,1974, internal report M 116). Especially
in the construction of PV-loops and the subsequent computation of stroke-
work it is essential to have interpolated signal values at disposal,
because the pressure and volume curves exhibit fast changes at different
time intervals. Therefore, the smoothing of the P(t) and V(t) curves precedes the plotting of the loop and the calculation of the area enclosed.

As shown in Fig. 9.5., M different quantities Q (LVV, LV- and aortic
pressure, aortic flow, *etc.*) of N heartbeats are processed, I being a
counting index. The elapsed time intervals are called RTA and RTB consecutively; if RTA becomes equal to or greater than RTB, the latter is
substituted as a new RTA, and the data values read are assigned to one
heartbeat (loop 5-2 in the diagram). These data values of all M quantities (loop 8-6) are submitted to the cubic spline function smoothing
procedure as described by REINSCH (1967), resulting in a set of four coefficients A through D with the beat index I. From these, interpolated
values of the quantities Q (M,N) may be calculated. Not shown in the
figure is the extensive overlay structure, necessary because of the limited memory space as mentioned in section IX.2. After the procedure
has been completed for all data belonging to one file (loop 11-1), the

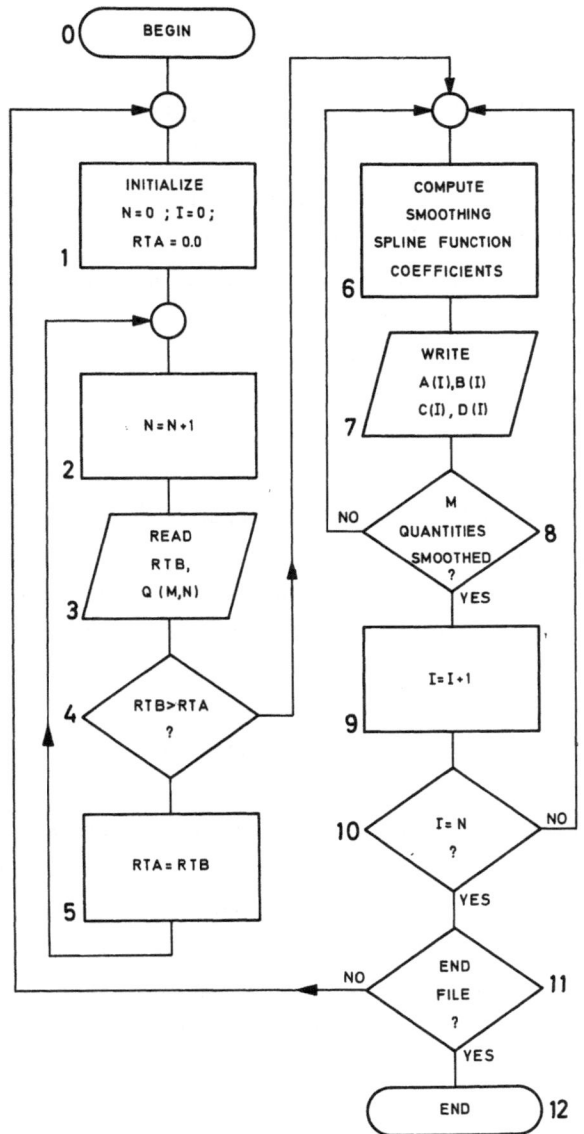

Fig. 9.5 Flow-Diagram of Smoothing Procedure

plotting programs use the interpolated values upon request of the operator.

5.2. Interactive_pseudo-threedimensional_presentation

To judge contraction patterns on a visual basis, a pseudo-threedimensional presentation of the ventricle under investigation may be required. The contour data are made available in the tape "B" structure for this purpose. With the help of the relevant geometric model, a set of surface coordinates can be reconstructed as shown in Fig. 9.6. (steps 1-2). The operator may choose the axis direction and the rotational position of the ventricle by introducing the three relevant angles in the orthogonal coordinate system. The surface is positioned accordingly by orthonormal transformation (steps 3-4). Hereby, the input buffer is overlayed by the output data. The object is cut into seven slices, perpendicular to the line connecting the viewer's eye and the center of the object. Each surface point is assigned an intensity modulation value corresponding to the slice it belongs to. The intensity is diminishing from the front to the back (step 5). Next, a perspective view is introduced (step 6) according to COULAM (1972). The result is displayed on a TV-monitor by means of a scan-converter output device, and judged for the details desired. If desired, the picture is refined by background suppression; this is realized by filling in the surface with small triangles. In the core image of the display device it is decided which points belong to the fore or background by comparing their z-modulation. Finally a fishing-net picture is derived, containing only the foreground lines (step 9). The result is displayed on the monitor; a polaroid picture can be taken from the scan converter memory tube, or a recording of the videosignal on the videodisk can be executed (step 10). If desired, the result can also be plotted. In this case, the z-modulation effect is omitted (steps 11-12). Steps 3 through 12 and 1 through 12 can be repeated upon command, until the clinician has obtained the additional information essential to his diagnostic procedure.

(Programme developed by G. Rol).

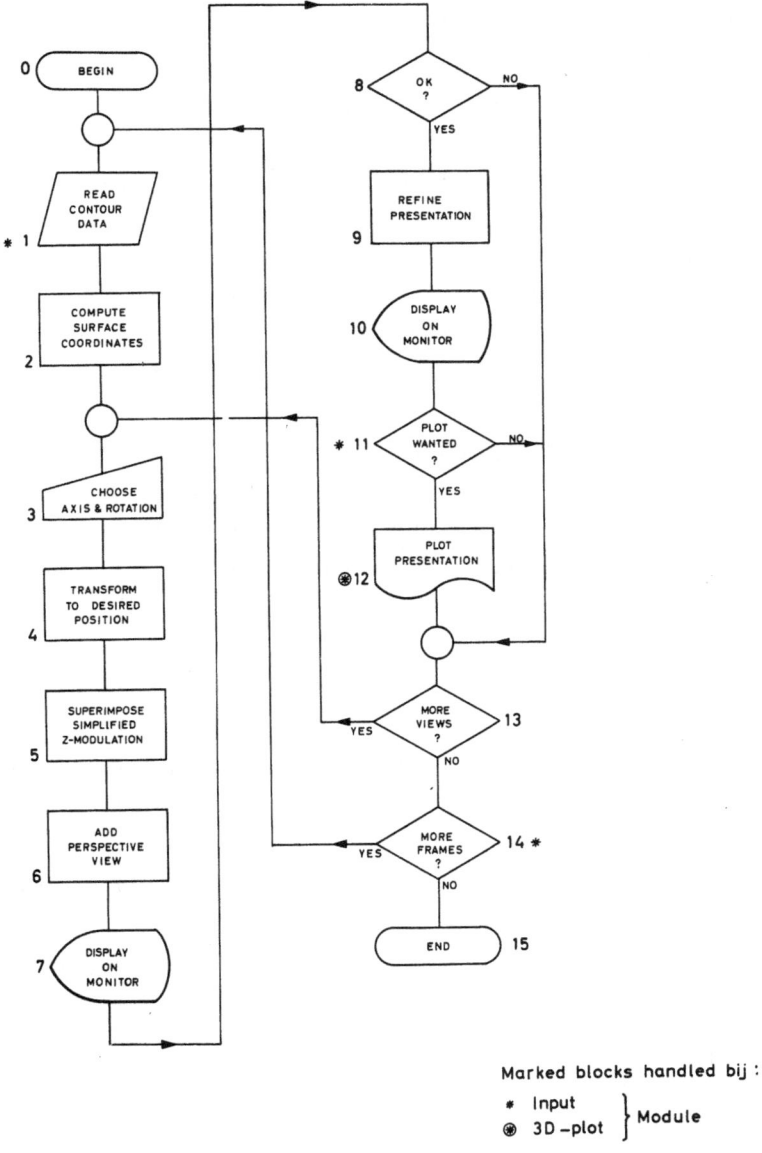

Fig. 9.6 Flow-Diagram of Interactive Pseudo-3D Presentation

5.3. Pseudo-threedimensional plotting programme

Some of the views, obtained according to the procedure described above, may require a hard-copy for filing with the patient's status. For this purpose, a plotting programme has been developed. The computed surface may be plotted as a projection on a plane, in every desired position. The method is depicted as a flow diagram in Fig. 9.7. This presentation requires the selection of the relative position of the body to the eye, the creation of a perspective and the depression of the "hidden" surfaces, formed by points of which the connection lines with the eye intersect another part of the surface. Our method for the description of the reconstructed LV-surface allows the use of a simple programme for the problem last mentioned. We start to compute the positions of all points projected on the plane with the slice that is nearest to that point of the axis which has the smallest distance to the eye. The points of this slice form a first region; the points of the next slice which fall within it are not seen. The other points together with the first region form a second one, which determines the visibility of the points of the following slices *etc.*

The equivalent diameters $\{x_i\}$ and $\{y_i\}$ as determined by the "VOLUM" module as quadrilateral projection lines, are read from tape "B". The parameters β and γ, determining the LV-axis spatial direction, the parameter ψ giving the rotational position around this axis and the indicator of contraction phase, θ, are read from this tape too. The set of indices of irregularity, α_i, specified by these parameters, are read in, as well as the corresponding array of cylindrical coordinates describing the general LV-shape (steps 1-4). The spatial model is placed in the same position as the ventricle at hand, and its sections with a set of planes through both X-ray foci and main axis dividing points are computed, as described in section IX.4. The individual centers of gravity, CGR_i, and areas, A_i, of these sections, are computed. The resulting section contours are expressed in polar coordinates and submitted to harmonic analysis, yielding HARM = $\{a'_n, b'_n\}_i$. With the help of the α_i

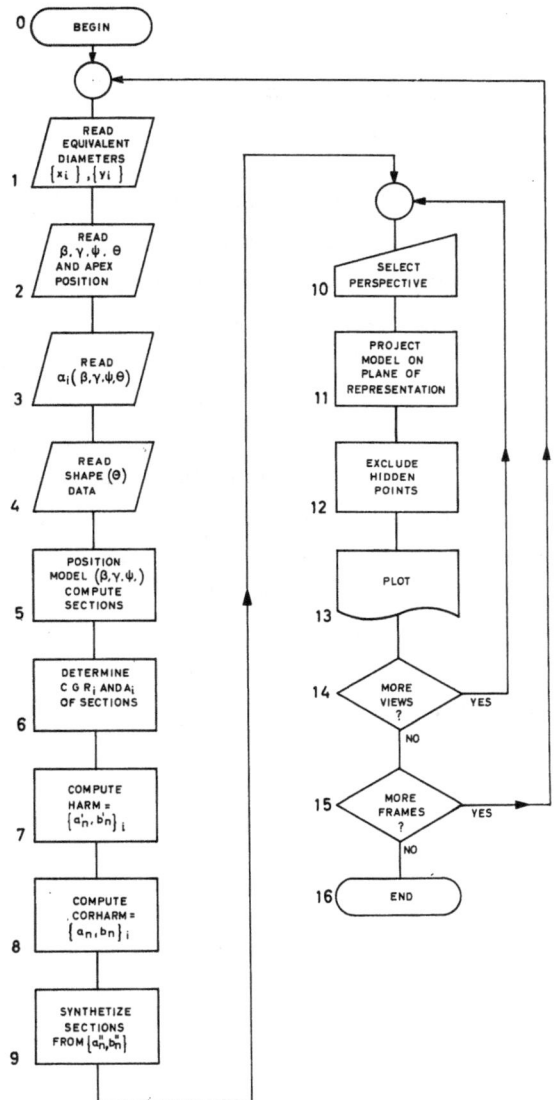

Fig. 9.7 Flow-Diagram of Pseudo-3D Plotting Program

and A_i, the FOURIER coefficients are transformed to

$$a_n = \frac{a_n'}{2} \sqrt{\frac{\alpha_i \, x_i \, y_i}{A_i}}; \quad b_n = \frac{b_n'}{2} \sqrt{\frac{\alpha_i \, x_i \, y_i}{A_i}} \quad \ldots \ldots \ldots \ldots (9.1)$$

thus a set of slices is constructed, adding up to the volume of the ventricle as calculated before (steps 5-8). From $\{a_n, b_n\}_i$, a set $\{a_n'', b_n''\}_i$ is computed by a dispersion-weighted transformation into a coefficient-configuration space, bringing the resynthetized contours back as much as possible into the quadrilateral cross sections (step 9). From a set of options, the desired viewing angles, eye position, and image plane, are selected by the operator. According to these parameters, the model is projected to the plane of representation. The "hidden points" are computed and omitted from the presentation. In this computation, use is made of the representation of the ventricle in slices, resulting in the simplified algorithm described above (steps 10-12).

After the projection has been plotted, more views of the same ventricle or of other frames may be selected (loops 14-10 and 15-1).

(Programmed by J. Heethaar).

146

6. Special Programs

Besides the software, needed for the calculations in the preceding sections, some special programs have been used for several purposes.

The "indices of irregularity" described in section VI.4, have been obtained by planimetry of casts, sliced perpendicularly to their main axis. In order to produce data relevant to other projection directions, mechanical division of the same casts would have been necessary (HEINT-ZEN 1974, LANGE, 1973). To obviate this, the contours of the individual slices from the same casts as used for the planimetry have been digitized, so that a pointwise description of the LV cavities resulted. From these data, the sections with planes subtending different angles with respect to the ventricular axis have been determined. From these, the "indices of irregularity" have been computed as the mean value of 12 ED-casts and 2 ES-casts respectively. The dimensions of dogs' heart casts allowed the blocks of clear plastic into which the casts had been embedded to be fraised in such a way, that slices of the size of 5x5 cm were obtained after mechanical sawing (see Fig. 6.2). By means of a slide projector and a TV-camera, the contours could easily by redrawn by the light-pen on a monitor. A slight modification of the software for contour entering served for introducing any new geometric model required.

The contour description programme is explained by Fig. 9.8. The contour and axis data are read from tape file A (Fig. 9.2), and corrected according to section IX.3. After the center of gravity of the "mass points" of each contour has been calculated, these points are represented in polar coordinates. By well-known numerical techniques, the FOURIER coefficients of the functions $r(\phi)$ are obtained. According to the mean values of the zero-order coefficients, a perpendicular search method is executed (steps 6-11), until the maximum "signal power" is contained in these coefficients. Thus, a set of new functions $r(\phi)$ is obtained, with respect to the new origin. Next, intervals of interest (ϕ_1, ϕ_2) can be chosen by the operator. The corresponding pieces of the contours to be compared are next described by a set of TSCHEBYCHEFF coefficients, c_k, the mean and standard deviation of which can be computed. These, as well as the corresponding quantities of the parameters of the axes, constitute the basis of comparison between groups of observers. Individual contours can be compared with the "mean contour" and "mean axis" of the group of experienced observers, which are taken as references.

The deviation of each individual contour from the "mean contour" may be judged visually (step 20), and expressed in the "relative absolute error" number according to Fig. 7.2. The data prepared as described above may next be submitted to Analysis of Variance, according to the aspects we may wish to investigate.

(Programme developed by J. Heethaar).

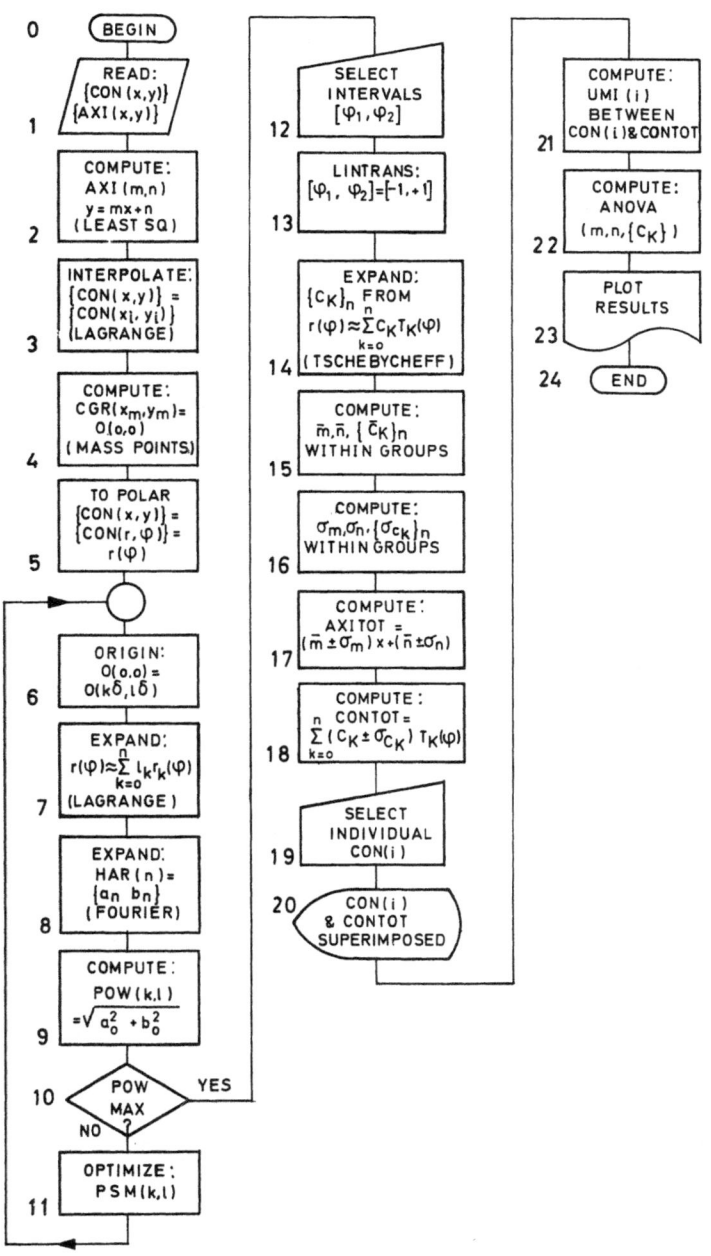

Fig. 9.8 Flow-Diagram of Contour Description Program

X. IN VIVO TESTS

1. *Introduction*

In addition to an analysis of error sources and their influence on the
accuracy of the result as will be given in Chapter XI, *in vivo* experiments are necessary. Besides the overall testing of the system, especially of the time programming by microcomputer, the effects of the geometric
model fit and the interindividual variability have to be established in
the real situation. During "steady state" of the circulation under controlled circumstances--especially with a constantly paced rhythm--thermo-
dilution gives a measure for the cardiac output (from which the stroke
volume can be derived by dividing through the heart rate) with a coefficient of variation of 4.3% (VAN DER WERF,1965). During this procedure,
an electromagnetic flow meter can be calibrated, so that the unknown
aortic lumen, haematocrit and other factors may be accounted for.
In this way, stroke volume may also be established with varying heart
rate. Although the blood flow into the coronary arteries escapes measure-
ment-–and this error may be estimated to be about 3% of mean flow--in
determining stroke volume it may be neglected because the maximum coronary flow occurs well after the end of the ventricular systole.

Several circuits have been described for integrating the signal of an electromagnetic flowmeter during each heartbeat. TEMPLES (1969) makes use of either the flow signal itself or of the left-ventricular pressure to control the integration period.

CALVERT (1973) employs the pacemaker signal for this purpose during controlled heart rate. The method chosen by us is an improvement of the design of DIJKEMA (1973), which features automatic zero adjustment and beat-to-beat mean flow computation. For our purpose, a sample-and-hold circuit is added to keep the integrator input signal at a constant value during the stimulation pulse. This has been proved necessary as the flow signal is distorted by the stimulation current causing a voltage across the measuring electrodes. The effect can be diminished by bipolar stimulation, for which specially-made electrodes are used.

For the kind of experiment described, open-chest surgery is necessary, but survival of the animal is not mandatory to the experimental results. According to one of the "Guiding Principles in the Care and Use of Animals", approved by the Council of the American Physiologic Society[')]

"Where the study does not require recovery from anesthesia, the animal must be killed in a human manner at the conclusion of the observations.",

the animal should be spared the suffering during recovery and an acute experiment is indicated. This allows the opportunity to use the sacrificed dogs' hearts for preparing casts during a well-defined state of contracture as described in section VI.3. Thus, comparing of *in vivo* and *in vitro* results of the same heart becomes possible without the need of many experimental animals. Besides, in the case of acute experiments the total amount of contrast material to be administered is not as limited as in the case of survival. This means that it can be chosen according to the image quality desired and the image recording capacity of the the videodisk, and that extensive measurement results are obtained from each animal. Measuring stroke volume is the principal purpose of the experiments, the determination of PV-loops and stroke work being secundary.

[')]Published in each number of the Amer. J. Physiol.

2. *Materials and Methods*

In five unpremedicated beagle dogs, weighing 9 to 11 kg (average 10 kg), anesthesia was induced with 25 mg per kg of pentothal (Nesdonal ®) intravenously, and maintained with 1 mg per kg and per hour of methadone (Symoron ®) and 0,25 mg per kg and per hour of dehydrobenzperidol (Droperidol ®) per infusion. Under capnographic control the respiration was kept at 4 to 4.5% CO_2 ET with a closed thorax by using 50% O_2 and 50% N_2O. The advantages of this procedure are that anesthesia is light, analgesia is strong, and that the heart rate has a low value (70-100 beats per minute) which is essential to our artificial stimulation programme. Furthermore, the circulation appeared to remain very stable.

Thoracotomy was performed, and a pair of stimulating electrodes (1mm ⌀ platinum eyelets) were sewn on to the right auricle. An electromagnetic flow probe of suitable diameter was placed around the ascending aorta. Then the thorax was closed air-tight using water-seal drainage to obtain a normal intrathoracic pressure. For measuring left-ventricular pressure a Miller microtip No. 8F catheter was introduced *via* one of the carotid arteries. The right femoral artery served for inserting a No. 7F Cordis pigtail angiographic catheter, to be connected to a Cordis Mark II contrast injector. In order to perform thermodilution, a thermistor-tip catheter (Swan-Ganz, type 93-113-7F) was placed in the pulmonary artery *via* the right femoral vein. About 7 ml of cold saline solution was injected in the *vena cava inferior*. The concentration-time curve as well as its time integral were obtained from a thermodilution unit, built by the clinic's electronics department, adapted for the dogs' cardiac output range. All relevant electric signals were recorded on magnetic tape (AMPEX FR 1300), papertape, as well as on "Anacor"channels. The cradle was placed in the 67° RAO position according to BENTIVOGLIO (1972), while the dogs were immobilized with a vacuum-fixation cushion (VAN DIEREN,1973) and rubber bands.

After these preparations, the experiment was carried out automatically at the command of the timing system implemented on the microcomputer described in section III.4.

3. *Results*.

In the sections II.5, VI.5, and VII.4 several technical properties of our system have been already mentioned. The results of the *in vivo* tests given here determine its feasibility in the real situation.

The time-programming system as described in section III.4 proved also to be a time-saver. After the surgical procedure, the measurements could be performed systematically and quickly. The facility of direct replay of the recorded images--in motion and as individual still pictures--in their original form or after subtraction, made direct visual judgement easy. The Vidicor signals, indicating the recent past, provided a good insight into the ventricular function in combination with the pictural information.

In this section two types of results will be presented. Firstly, from one and the same set of contours and axes left-ventricular volumes have been computed according to DODGE's area-length method, the CHAPMAN stack-of-elliptical-cylinders procedure, and our index of irregularity method. The corresponding scatter diagrams of Fig. 10.1 and 10.2 present the data obtained, separately for the ES and ED-volumes as different indices of irregularity have been used by us in both cases. Secondly, the method developed by us has been checked against simultaneous electromagnetic flow measurements. The stroke volumes obtained as the difference between the angiographically determined end-diastolic and end-systolic volumes have been compared with those computed as the time integral of the aortic flow. Because of the low sampling frequency of the system, the pictures from which the LVV has been calculated do in general not coincide exactly with these physiological instants. The correct time intervals for the integration of the flow could be reconstructed, however, from the recorded trigger signals for the X-ray installation. The scatter diagram of Fig. 10.3 shows the values measured.

With respect to the statistical evaluation of our data, the following comments can be made:
The comparison between our values for the stroke volume and those obtained from integrated flow measurements show a **reasonable correlation**

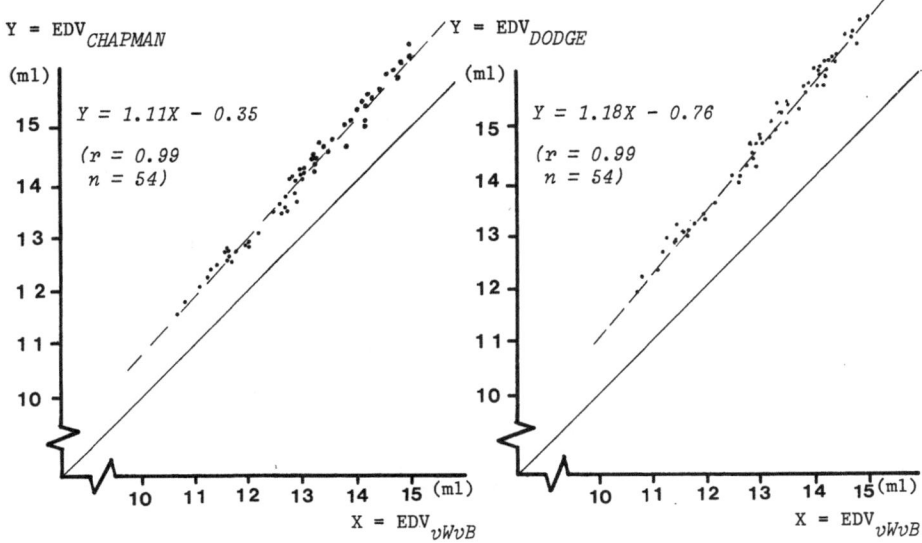

Fig. 10.1 *Comparison of Geometric Models In Vivo (EDV)*

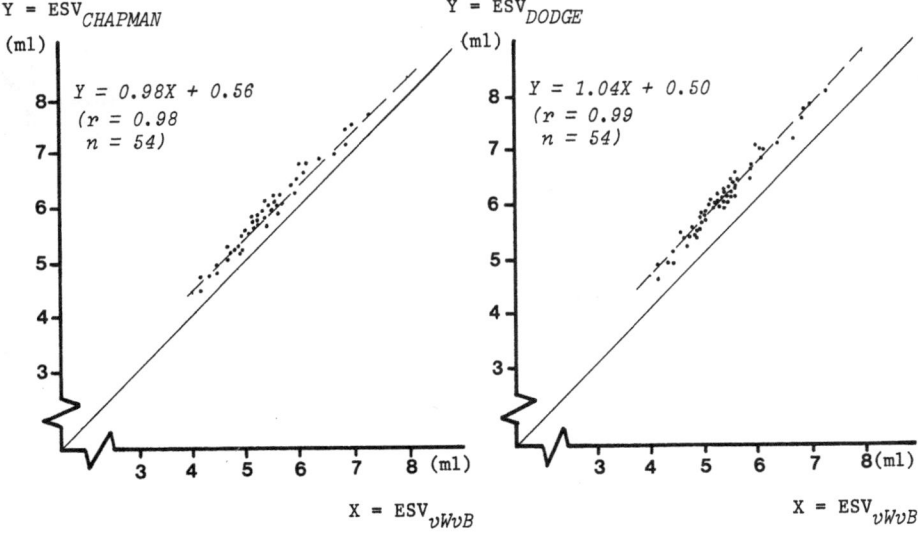

Fig. 10.2 *Comparison of Geometric Models In Vivo (ESV)*

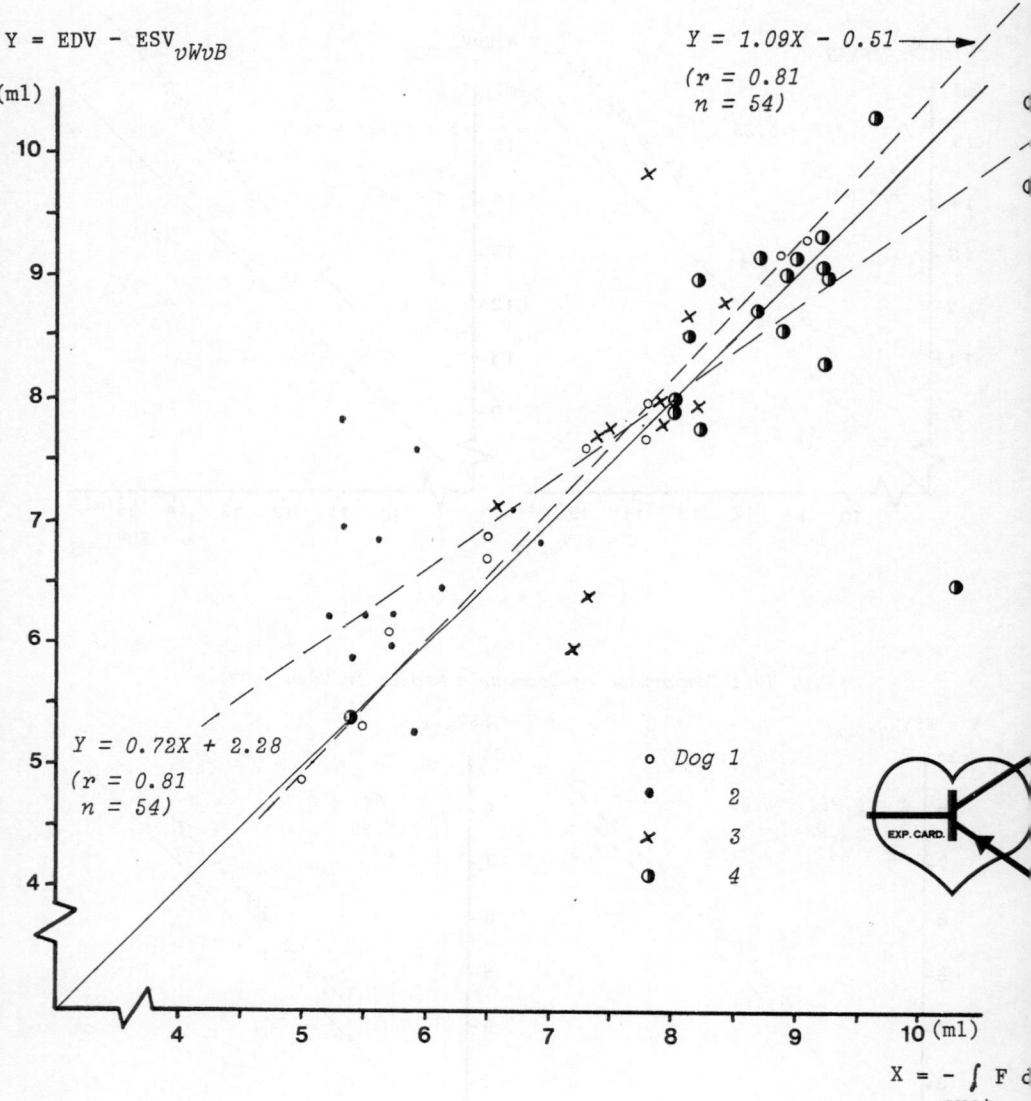

Fig. 10.3 Comparison of SV by Angiographic and EM-flow Methods

156

(Fig. 10.3). Moreover, the values indicate a good relation, which should be noted because the two techniques are totally independent. It is felt that with regard to the statistical uncertainties as expressed in the confidence limits given, it can be concluded that both methods give a good estimate of the stroke volume. The discrepancies which show up in some points could not be traced to a specific error source. The theoretical standard deviation, see Chapter XI, is of the order of 1 ml for the SV. The EM-flowmeter measurements as described are estimated to have a standard deviation of the order of 10%.

Furthermore, a comparison between our model and those of CHAPMAN and DODGE has been made, using the same contours (Figs. 10.1 and 10.2). If our volumes were taken as the independent variable, within the range of volumes measured, regression lines were adapted based on the assumptions of linearity and normal distribution, which, of course, are not warranted in this material. The regression lines for EDV and ESV deviate clearly from equality, and indicate an overestimation of the two models in all cases. For the stroke volumes both methods come to a rather close agreement, but also here the fit is not too good.

The results, plotted together in the scatter diagrams, have been obtained from four dogs. As experimental conditions will have varied from dog to dog, the data have been analyzed separately for these cases also. The regression equations and correlation coefficients have been tabulated in section XIII.3, showing high correlation coefficients in the cases a, b and c_1. In comparing the stroke volumes, the data according to both methods have been chosen to act as the independent variable, yielding two regression lines. Here, 95% confidence limits for the correlation coefficient have been computed after applying FISHER's z-transformation (ZAR,1974). For the regression coefficients the t-test has been used.

In conclusion, the ED and ES-volume measurements according to different models from the same set of basic data show great consistency. The stroke volume measurements differ strongly from case to case. The results of dog No. 1 are quite satisfactory; dog No. 4 exhibits widely scattered points.

XI. UNCERTAINTY ANALYSIS

1. *Introduction*

The veracious experimenter must provide the reader with some measure of
the reliability of his results. Ideally, this reliability should be
assured by the use of statistics applied to multiple-sample experiments. Unfortunately, estimating all the uncertainties by repetition
is often not practical. So, in the case of single-sample experiments
another method for the description and analysis of uncertainties has
to be used. For a single observation, the "error", which is the difference between the--unknown--true and the observed value, is a certain
--though again unknown--number. But the "uncertainty", the estimate of
the error, may vary considerably depending upon the particular circumstances of the observation. The "result" is obtained by making corrections to or calculations with "variables", *i.e.* the basic quantities observed directly. The recorded values of the variables are called "data".
The way in which uncertainties in the variables affect the uncertainties in the result is called "propagation of uncertainty". In single-
sample experiments the statements of reliability will inevitably be
partly based on estimates, since by definition statistics cannot
be applied to all the errors. A method for estimating and

for calculating the propagation of these uncertainties into the results has been given by KLINE (1953) and will be followed in this chapter.

Analyzing the measurement procedure leads to the conclusion that the derivation of an analytic expression for the result as a function of all conceivable independent variables is not feasible. Therefore, in section 2 of this Chapter error sources, leading to uncertainty intervals in relevant variables, will be discussed separately. The sensitivity of the result for these variables, though formally to be expressed as partial derivatives, will be established by computer simulation. To this end, the effects of deliberately induced variations have been computed for some important cases. Next, estimates will be given for the corresponding uncertainty intervals as expected from system component properties and/or experience. Then, conclusions may be drawn on the propagation of uncertainty in a linear approximation to be explained in section 3. Both the maximum absolute error to be expected and the probable error under the assumption of normally distributed variables can be calculated from the data gathered. Thus a quantitative insight can be given into the factors determining the reliability of the result.

One aspect, however, will escape our analysis. As long as we lack an extensive collection of casts of pathological cases, the degree of fit of the geometric model to the patient's ventricle will preclude an exact correspondance. The possibility of obtaining extra information on the shape of the ventricle under investigation has already been discussed in section II.4, (JOHNSON,1973), but the equipment required is not available at this time.

2. *Uncertainty Intervals for Relevant Variables.*

In this analysis, the following variables have been considered relevant, as will be discussed below.

a. The distances L_1, L_2, D_1, D_2, are determined from the steel measuring bands as described in section II.4. The mechanical stability of the supports in combination with the observational error of the bands gives rise to an uncertainty of ± 1 mm. In this quantity the uncertainty in the location of the focal spot with respect to the arrow indicating its position on the X-ray tube housing, as well as possible variations in the focus location on the tube anode, have been included. Thus, the distances used in the calculation of the magnification factor may suffer from uncertainty intervals w_1 through w_4, which have a value of about 2 mm.

b. As described in section IX.3, the ventricular axis is reconstructed in its true spatial position and dimensions from axes drawn in the projection planes and their intercepts with the contours. One set of independent variables is constituted by the parameters determining these axes relative to the coordinate systems in the two projection planes. The variability in these parameters is concluded from the standard deviations thereof as computed in section VII.4. These four variables have been assigned uncertainty intervals w_5, w_7 for the slopes and w_6, w_8 for the ordinate intercepts. The influence of the axis lengths will be estimated separately, as these are determined by the axes and the contours together (w_9, w_{10}).

c. As can be seen in Figs 7.5 and 7.6, the relation between the contour descriptors and the sets of contour diameters x_i and y_i is a difficult one. Therefore, the uncertainty intervals of these diameters have been determined for the average values of three equal groups of diameters corresponding with one-third of the number of division points on the ventricular axis. This yields the uncertainty intervals w_{11} through w_{17}.

d. In an intricate combination, the variables w_1 through w_{12} give the basic input data which are used to reconstruct a digitized *replica* of the ventricle at hand if the geometric model chosen by us is applied. This model is given by the relevant set of indices of irregularity α_i and the FOURIER descriptors $\{a_n, b_n\}_i$ of the shape of the i slices into which the model has been divided. This gives too large a number of variables for our purpose, therefore a data compression technique has been applied. The α_i-curves as depicted in Fig. 6.4 are described by the average of six successive equal groups of α_i, yielding w_{17} through w_{22} according to the interindividual variability of the casts on which the model has been based, and which has been depicted as vertical bars in the figure mentioned. The shape descriptors are used only in the case of constructing a pseudo-3D presentation, and thus need not be considered here.

Table 11.1 in section XIII.3 contains the numerical values of the uncertainty intervals of the variables discussed above. The degree to which their influence is propagated into the result of our volume calculations will be discussed in the following section.

3. Propagation of Uncertainty

Let the result R be a function of n independent variables v_i, in which variations Δv_i occur which give rise to a variation ΔR in the result

$$R \pm \Delta R = R(v_1 \pm \Delta v_1, v_2 \pm \Delta v_2, \ldots, v_n \pm \Delta v_n) \quad \ldots \ldots (11.1)$$

Expanding this equation in a TAYLOR series, subtracting the corresponding value $R(v_1, v_2, \ldots, v_n)$, and discarding the higher-order terms yields the following expression for the absolute error

$$\Delta R = \sum_{i=1}^{n} \left| \frac{\partial R}{\partial v_i} \Delta v_i \right| \quad \ldots \ldots \ldots \ldots \ldots \ldots \ldots \ldots (11.2)$$

If the independent variables v_i are each normally distributed, then the relation between the uncertainty intervals for the variables, w_i, and the interval for the result, w_R, giving the same odds for each of the variables and for the result, is

$$w_R = \left[\sum_{i=1}^{n} \left(\frac{\partial R}{\partial v_i} w_i \right)^2 \right]^{\frac{1}{2}} \quad \ldots \ldots \ldots \ldots \ldots \ldots \ldots (11.3)$$

which equation might be used directly as an approximation for calculating the uncertainty interval in the result. To this end, the uncertainty intervals, w_i, as specified in section XI-2, have to be confronted with the sensitivity of the result, $\partial R / \partial v_i$, for changes in the corresponding variables, v_i.

The absolute error, ΔR according to (11.2) as well as the uncertainty interval in the result, w_R according to (11.3) will both be calculated, assuming the requirements for the latter are fulfilled in approximation.

4. Uncertainty Interval in the Result.

The procedure for calculating the propagation of uncertainty intervals into the result as described in the preceding section requires the determination of the "sensitivity" $\partial R/\partial v_i$ of the result to these uncertainties. The complexity of the volume calculation procedure precludes computation in analytical form. Therefore, the sensitivities have been established by computer experiments. In a randomly chosen set of ES-input data, variations in the range of values as discussed in section XI.2 have been introduced one at a time, to determine the partial derivatives. It seems justified to assume that no singular points in the hyperplane $R(v_1, v_2, \dots, v_n)$ are present. An ES-case has been chosen because the influence of the uncertainty intervals in the set of indices of irregularity, α_i, proved greater than in end-diastole where the ventricular shape is smoother.

The values have been entered into Table 11.1 (Section XIII.3); from the last two columns of this table the conclusions may be drawn that the main sources of error are to be ascribed to the two lowest-numbered sets of contour diameters in both projections $(v_{11}, v_{12}, v_{14}, v_{15})$ as well as to the four lowest-numbered of the six parts of the model $(v_{17}$ through $v_{20})$.
As was only to be expected, the region of the aortic and mitral valves is the most difficult.
The maximum absolute error, ΔR, equals 1.3 ml and the uncertainty interval in the result to be expected, w_R = 0.4 ml in this worst-case analysis.
In the example we used, R = ESV_{vWvB} = 5.7 ml, so the probable error amounts to 7%, giving a useful estimate for judging the results of Fig. 10.3

XII. DISCUSSION

In the measurement system described in this thesis, several advanced techniques are applied to the quantitation of the left heart's pumping function. This introduces problems of instrumental as well as of methodological nature. As an X-ray installation is used as a part of the measurement installation, its properties have been investigated. The spatial image transfer characteristics of modern image intensifiers pose no principal problems, but the video part of the system may become a limiting factor. Central synchronization of the X-ray-television subsystem, phase-locked to the mains, is required in order to achieve well-determined radiation pulses. From section II.3. it is concluded that jitter in the synchronization is reflected in a frame-to-frame spatial displacement of picture elements of the order of 0.1 mm. This effect can be neglected in comparison with the accuracy of the LV-contour determination. In videosubtraction it results in a "shift unsharpness" which is rather small compared with other sources of error. Raising the master oscillator frequency from 10 MHz to about 500 MHz can solve this problem; it should be considered in combination with the properties of all other links in the TV-chain, especially of the recording/reproducing part and of the electronics used for manipulation of the videosignal. The temporal image transfer characteristics as shown in Fig. 2.7 determine the limitations in the depiction of small, fast moving structures, as well as the effect of the 50 Hz frame frequency. As each image sample is composed of two such frames, which interlaced give a complete field, the sampling frequency can be doubled at the cost of halving the number of scanning lines. Our system has been designed for 50 images per second; this frequency can only be exploited, however, if the manufacturer of the video-disk can provide double the rotation speed, which is not yet the case by now. Should this modification be realized, isochronous coupling of the cinecameras to the central synchronization unit will be a further step toward a more versatile angiography installation, apart from the video-tape archivation aspects mentioned in section V.5.

A methodological aspect of our system concerns the contrast medium injection procedure. In order to gain as much information as possible from the catheterization, the administration of the medium has to be performed in as many portions as possible. Because the injection pressure is limited for reasons of safety and to avoid mechanically induced extra-systoles, the injector has to be programmed, especially in the case of irregular RR-intervals. The intricate time programming system which controls the total procedure may therefore justly be called the heart of the installation. In order to "synchronize" the patient with the measurement, artificial stimulation is required. Although this may limit the categories of patients for which the system is useful, the method will give much more quantitative insight in the condition of those patients which are examined by clinical stimulation. In that case, angiograms can be taken at predetermined beats, which follow the synchronization pattern but are embedded in a sequence of stimulation pulses, chosen on other grounds, *e.g.* artificial atrial fibrillation.

As has been shown in sections II.4 and VI.5, the facility of semi-continuous correction for the projective enlargement in a biplane installation has been exploited as much as possible. Calibration is simple and accurate; shortly the positions of the X-ray foci and image-intensifier input screen centers will be measured automatically and coupled to the Digicor counter inputs. The geometric model as proposed in section VI.4 makes use of the true position of the ventricular axis in space, applies an individual magnification correction factor to each elementary volume ("slice"), and is based on a general shape of the ven-

tricle for various cases. At the cost of loss of accuracy, however, the
model might be used in a monoplane installation, if an average position
of the ventricle can be established, *e.g.* by making one extra picture
with the cradle rotated or with a mobile second X-ray installation. A
new set of "indices of irregularity" together with a determination of
the ventricular axis position should be established in that case.

Determination of the ventricular shadow contours is one of the main
problems in quantitative angiocardiography. In our opinion, the a priori
information to be given by the trained operator should be included to
obtain the maximum benefit of the pictures. Videosubtraction has been
performed successfully, and provides a picture which is free from many
disturbing details. Besides, it can serve as the basis for other procedures, *e.g.* determination of the ventricular "slice" areas from their
biplane density profiles, or semi-automatic contour detection in which
the operator only has to choose templates for the difficult regions of
the contour, while the remaining part is determined on the basis of local density gradients.

The integrated information recording facilities of the system obviate
many labourious manual tasks, and reduce human errors by direct coupling
of the read-out subsystems to the computer. Its main drawback is the
sampling frequency of the analog signals, which is equal to the image
frequency. Thus, fast phenomena will be missed. Special investigations,
e.g. deriving contractility indices from the LV-pressure, cannot be performed with the signal samples. Such indices, however, reflect a general
condition, and in most cases identification with individual X-ray images
will not be required.

The modular structure of the software package guarantees a flexibility, needed to adapt the system to the clinician's needs. Coupling the
Digicor to the microcomputer which governs the measurement will result
in a fault-free record keeping; linking it to the PDP-15 computer during
the evaluation procedure can provide the operator with a simple set of
actions to be performed. These facilities are still under development,
and will be implemented in close collaboration with the medical staff.

The propagation of uncertainties due to several independent error sources gives insight in the factors determining the accuracy of the volume measurement. A possible solution for the main source of error, the drawing of the LV-contours in the region of the valves, is a systematical training program for operators. Discussions among various observers during our experiments lead to the conclusion, that the judgement should be supplemented by knowledge of how the contours drawn are used for reconstruction of the ventricular cavity by our model. The already-mentioned article by RAPHAEL (1974) might prove helpful in this program. Thus, questions as to whether to include certain structures when drawing contours might be answered satisfactorily. Only after this measuring the intraindividual variability of the observer is a useful method for establishing the error due to the man-machine part of the system.

The ever-remaining source of error is the degree of correspondence between the patient's ventricular shape and the geometric model used. Thus a remaining task is to establish sets of $\alpha_i(\theta)$, in which the parameter θ denotes a certain class of hearts. Data on human ventricular casts according to LANGE (1974) as well as the casts themselves have been made available to us by the courtesy of this author[']. Thus models adapted to patients will be introduced in the system presently, after which clinical use of it can be made. The computed worst-case probable error of about 7% indicates the justification of this introduction into the clinic.

[']Department of Pediatric Cardiology and Bioengineering, University Childrens' Hospital, Christian-Albrechts-University, Kiel, Federal Republic of Germany (Director: Prof.Dr.Med. P.H. Heintzen).

XIII. APPENDIX

1. Glossary

1.1 List_of_Symbols

a   Longitudinal dimension of X-ray focus; major axis of general ellipsoid

b   *(Suffix)*: Ball (in spherical model); minor axis of general ellipsoid

c   Volume concentration; *(suffix)*: contrast (in spherical model); minor axis of general ellipsoid

d   Distance; thickness of absorbing layer; diameter (in spherical model)

e   Base of natural logarithms

f   Temporal frequency; geometric magnification factor

h   Thickness of elementary slice in geometric model of left ventricular cavity

i   *(Suffix)*: index of natural numbers

j   *(Suffix)*: index of natural numbers; unit of imaginary numbers $(\sqrt{-1})$

k   Order of term in polynomial expansion

m   *(Suffix)*: centre of gravity of point masses; coefficient of direction in representation of straight line

n   Natural number (upper limit in summation of finite series); ordinate interception in representation of straight line; number of samples

o   *(Suffix)*: incident radiation

r   Coordinate in polar system, correlation coefficient (sample)

s   *(Suffix)*: spatial; *(suffix)*: scattered radiation; standard deviation (sample)

t   *(Suffix)*: temporal

v   Velocity; variable in measurement result

w   Uncertainty interval; *(Suffix)*: water (in spherical model)

x,y   Coordinates in orthogonal system
z

A	Area enclosed by ventricular shadow contour
C	Contrast in adjacent picture elements, defined in Fig. 4.2
D	Distance of X-ray tube focus to coordinate axis; thickness of absorbing layer; length of minor ellipsoid axis
E	Quantum energy
F	Planimetered area of heart shadow, flow
I	Intensity of radiation, signal current of vidicon/plumbicon
L	Distance of image-intensifier input screen to coordinate axis; length of ventricular main axis
O	Origin of coordinate system
P	L-ventricular pressure
R	Measurement result; radius of sphere
V	Volume; momentary value of videosignal
X,Y	Axes of orthogonal coordinate system
Z	Atomic number; axis of orthogonal coordinate system

AP	Anterio-posterior projection direction
BSA	Body surface area
EDV	End-diastolic volume
EF	Ejection fraction
EFS	Effective focal spot size
ESV	End-systolic volume
ET	End-tidal
HT	High-tension
LSF	Line-spread function
LVV	Left-ventricular cavity volume
MTF	Modulation transfer function
OTF	Optical transfer function
PSF	Point-spread function
SV	Stroke volume
SW	Stroke work

α,β,γ Angles in orthogonal coordinate system

ϵ Relative error

θ Index for type of heart in geometric model

μ Linear extinction coefficient

ν Spatial frequency

π Circumference-to-diameter ratio of circle

ρ Density, correlation coefficient (population)

σ Standard deviation (square root of variance), of population

τ Time; time constant; pulse duration

ϕ Coordinate in polar coordinate system

ψ Angle of rotation of the ventricular cavity around its main axis, measured counterclockwise from the middle of the intraventricular septum

Δ *(Operator)*: difference

Σ *(Operator)*: summation

a_i Weight fraction

a_n, b_n FOURIER coefficients of order n sine and cosine terms respectively

c_k TSCHEBYCHEFF coefficient of order k

l_k LANGRANGIAN polynomial of order k

x_i', y_i' Ventricular contour diameter pairs

ΔA_i Area of elementary slice of ventricular cavity

$S(\nu)$ Amplitude spectrum of spatial frequencies

$T_k(.)$ TSCHEBYCHEFF polynomial of the first kind and order k of argument

ΔV_i Volume of elementary slice of ventricular cavity

α_i Index of irregularity

$\bar{\mu}$ Effective linear extinction coefficient

μ/ρ Mass absorption coefficient

v *(Operator)*: unity (in VENN-diagram)

$\wedge$ *(Operator)*: intersection (in VENN-diagram)

dP/dt Time derivative of ventricular pressure

$\partial R/\partial v$ Partial derivative of result R with respect to variable v

1.2 List of Terms

Absorbed Dose: Amount of energy imparted by ionizing paticles and photons per unit of mass.

Afterload: Force to be developed by the individual myocardial fibers in order to meet the end-diastolic aortic pressure against which the left ventricle has to pump out.

Contour: Closed curve in the image plane defining the border of the LV-cavity shadow projection.

Contractility: Ability of the myocardium to exert force; the contractile state of the muscle fibers is reflected by their force-velocity-length relations. Sometimes the relative height of the FRANK-STARLING-curve is used as a measure.

Contrast: Difference in luminance of an object--or its pictural representation-- and the background divided by the mean brightness of both.

Drop-out: Imperfection in the recording/reproducing process of a videosignal on magnetic material due to the finite dimension of the head gap, thus precluding recording on all lines of a frame.

Ejection Fraction: Stroke volume expressed as a fraction of end-diastolic volume.

End-diastolic Volume: Volume of blood contained in the left-ventricular heart cavity at the occurrence of the R-wave in the electrocardiogram in lead II.

End-systolic Volume: Residual volume of blood contained in the left-ventricular cavity after completing of contraction.

Extra-systole: Premature contraction of the heart muscle; can be induced mechanically by catheter movement or fluid jet from contrast medium injection.

Field: Television picture of 625 lines formed by two interlacing frames.

Focus (X-ray-): Orthogonal projection of the bombarded area on the anode of an X-ray tube in the direction of the beam axis.

Frame: Television half-picture, composed of $312\frac{1}{2}$ lines. Intended for interlacing, may also be used as a seperate sample of the image.

Index: Circulatory parameter, divided by the body surface area to obtain interindividually comparable results.

Index of Irregularity: Ratio of the area to the product of diameters in an elementary slice of a model of the left-ventricular cavity. Its difference from $\pi/4$ indicates the irregularity in shape as compared with an ellipse.

Isoplanasy: Shift-invariance of transfer characteristics in--a part of--an imaging system.

Isotropy: Direction-invariance of transfer characteristics in--a part of--an imaging system, causing the point-spread-function to have rotational symmetry.

Latch: Digital buffer memory.

Line-spread Function: Response of an imaging system to a two-dimensional intensity impulse, generated by a line-shaped source.

Modulation: Difference of the maximum and minimum radiation intensity, as caused by a stationary or moving test object, divided by the sum of these.

Modulation Transfer Function: Modulus of the normalized optical transfer function, with two spatial and one temporal frequencies as arguments.

Morphometry: Technique in which a pseudo-three-dimensional picture of a cavity is generated by a computer, based on shadow contours and a geometric model.

Multiplexer: Analog or digital switching circuit, connecting several inputs to one output at the command of a separate signal.

Object Spectrum: FOURIER transform of the intensity distribution in a picture according to a given direction.

Optical Transfer Function: FOURIER transform of the line-spread function of an imaging system.

Patch: Two-dimensional region in which an imaging system possesses shift-invariant transmission properties.

Point-spread Function: Response of an imaging system to an intensity impulse, generated by a point-shaped source.

Preload: Initial values of myocardial fiber lengths or tensions in the relaxed state, as reflected by the end-diastolic volume of the left ventricle.

Strain: Change in dimension relative to initial length.

Stress: Force per unit of area in a cross-section perpendicular to the force direction. Positive sign indicates dilation, negative sign indicates compression.

Stroke Volume: Net volume of blood expelled by the left ventricle during one stroke; difference between successive end-diastolic and end-systolic volumes if no regurgitation takes place.

Stroke Work: Net external work delivered by the myocard during one stroke; difference between systolic and diastolic work as expressed by the area enclosed by the pressure-volume curve.

Subtraction: Technique for cancelling non-relevant details of an image by photographical or electronical means, using a second picture containing these details only.

Synchronization: Technique for ascertaining correspondence in time of events; especially the visual components in television by using a well-defined pulse pattern.

Videoangiocardiography: Technique for recording X-ray pictures of heart cavities, filled with radiopaque material, as videosignals.

Videometry: Technique in which measures are derived from images represented by videosignals.

Videosignal: Electric signal, representing images, consisting of a pulse pattern containing timing and level reference and parts reflecting the image brightness along scanning lines.

2. *Derivations*

2.1 Calculation of the Number of Contrast Medium Fractions

As proposed by SNEEK (1971, internal report M82), the ventricle within
the thorax is modelled by a sphere of radius R, filled with a volume
concentration c of contrast medium with a linear extinction coefficient
μ_c, embedded in a flat layer of thickness D of water-like substance
with a linear extinction coefficient μ_w. The mixture within the ball
then has a linear extinction coefficient

$$\mu_2 = c\mu_c + (1 - c)\mu_w \quad \ldots \ldots \ldots \ldots \ldots \ldots \ldots (13.1)$$

If monochromatic radiation is assumed, the intensity I(x) of the outgoing radiation as a function of the distance x from the center amounts
to (Fig. 13.1)

$$I_2(x) = I_0\, e^{-\{\mu_2 2\sqrt{R^2-x^2} + \mu_1(D-2\sqrt{R^2-x^2})\}} \quad \ldots \ldots \ldots (13.2^a)$$

for $0 \overset{\leq}{=} |x| \overset{\leq}{=} R$, and to

$$I_1(x) = I_0\, e^{-\mu_1 D} \quad \ldots \ldots \ldots \ldots \ldots \ldots (13.2^b)$$

for $|x| \overset{\geq}{=} R$; I_0 being the incident radiation intensity.

The contrast C(x) between the border of the sphere with radius x and
its surrounding, ($|x| \overset{\geq}{=} R$), defined according to the spatial modulation
depth, amounts to (JAEGER,1969)

$$C(x) = \frac{I_2(x) - I_1(x)}{I_1(x) + I_2(x)} = \frac{\Delta I(x)}{2I_1(x) + \Delta I(x)} \quad \ldots \ldots \ldots \ldots (13.3^a)$$

With $\Delta I(x) = I_2(x) - I_1(x)$ $\ldots \ldots \ldots \ldots \ldots \ldots (13.3^b)$

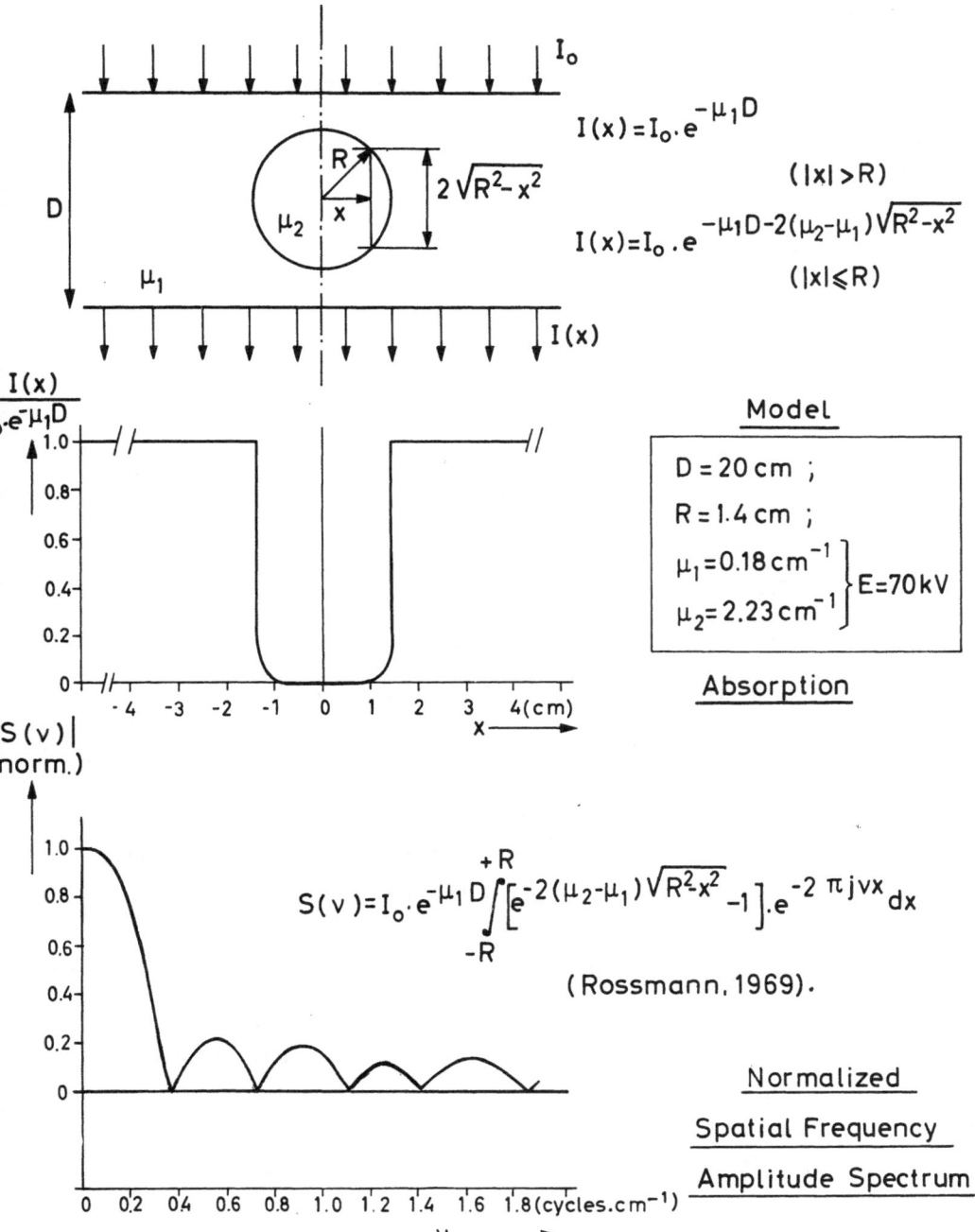

$$I(x) = I_o \cdot e^{-\mu_1 D} \quad (|x| > R)$$

$$I(x) = I_o \cdot e^{-\mu_1 D - 2(\mu_2 - \mu_1)\sqrt{R^2 - x^2}} \quad (|x| \leqslant R)$$

Model

D = 20 cm ;
R = 1.4 cm ;
$\mu_1 = 0.18\,\mathrm{cm}^{-1}$
$\mu_2 = 2.23\,\mathrm{cm}^{-1}$ } E = 70 kV

Absorption

$$S(v) = I_o \cdot e^{-\mu_1 D} \int_{-R}^{+R} \left[e^{-2(\mu_2 - \mu_1)\sqrt{R^2 - x^2}} - 1 \right] \cdot e^{-2\pi j v x} dx$$

(Rossmann, 1969).

Normalized
Spatial Frequency
Amplitude Spectrum

Fig. 13.1 Simplified Absorption Model

175

$$C(x) \simeq \frac{\Delta I(x)}{2I_1(x)} \text{ , if it may be assumed that } \frac{\Delta I(x)}{I_1(x)} \ll 1 \quad \ldots \ldots (13.4)$$

Also: $\quad \frac{1}{2}\ln \frac{I_2(x)}{I_1(x)} = \frac{1}{2}\ln\{1 + \frac{\Delta I(x)}{I_1(x)}\} \simeq \frac{\Delta I(x)}{2I_1(x)} \simeq C(x) \quad \ldots \ldots (13.5^a)$

And: $\quad \frac{1}{2}\ln \frac{I_2(x)}{I_1(x)} = (\mu_b - \mu_w)\sqrt{R^2-x^2} \quad \ldots \ldots \ldots (13.5^b)$

With: $\quad \mu_b - \mu_w = c(\mu_w - \mu_c) = c\Delta\mu \quad \ldots \ldots \ldots (13.6^a)$

and: $\quad \Delta\mu = \mu_w - \mu_c \quad \ldots \ldots \ldots \ldots (13.6^b)$

to be taken from table 3.2 (section XIII.4),we find:

$$C(x) \simeq c\Delta\mu\sqrt{R^2-x^2} = c\Delta\mu R\sqrt{1 - (x/R)^2} \quad \ldots \ldots \ldots (13.7)$$

The ratio x/R depends on the relative volume error ΔV we allow

$$\Delta V = \frac{\frac{3}{4}\pi R^3 - \frac{3}{4}\pi x^3}{\frac{3}{4}\pi R^3} = 1 - (x/R)^3 \quad \ldots \ldots \ldots \ldots (13.8)$$

$$x/R = (1 - \Delta V)^{1/3} \simeq 1 - \frac{\Delta V}{3} \text{ , if } \Delta V \ll 1 \quad \ldots \ldots \ldots (13.9)$$

Inserting this expression into (13.7) we obtain:

$$C(x) \simeq c\Delta\mu R\sqrt{\frac{2\Delta V}{3}} \quad \ldots \ldots \ldots \ldots (13.10)$$

This contrast of the primary radiation is diminished by the scattered radiation intensity I_s, which may be assumed to be uniformly distributed within the sphere and outside, because:

$$\left| \ln \frac{I_2(x) + I_s}{I_1(x) + I_s} \right| < \left| \ln \frac{I_2(x)}{I_1(x)} \right| \quad \ldots \ldots \ldots (13.11)$$

Under the assumption that the X-ray contrast is transformed linearly to the TV-monitor--which in general is not the case--it may be derived from SCHOBER (1966) that for a room illumination level of 10 cd.m^{-2} a ratio $\Delta I_{tot}/I_{tot} = 0.01$ should be taken.

In section III.2 it has already be assumed that the scattered radiation intensity $I_s = 4I_2$, so we find:

$$I_2(x)/I_1(x) = 0.95 \quad \text{and thus} \quad C(x) = 0.025 \ldots \ldots \ldots (13.12)$$

If a $\Delta V = 0.01$ is permitted, the allowable volume concentration may be calculated with R as a parameter.

Thereby, the dependence of $\Delta\mu$ on the quantum energy, E, as given in Table 3.2 (section XIII.4) has to be taken into account, with reference to the energy spectrum of the incident radiation, $dI_o(E)/dE$ for different tube voltages as shown in Fig. 13.2. [']

The definition of the effective linear extinction coefficient $\bar{\mu}$ according to SCHOKNECHT (1966) as mentioned in section III.2 has been used in a modified form, the spectrum being given in n discrete points:

$$\bar{\mu} = - \ln \frac{\sum\limits_{i=1}^{n} \dfrac{\Delta I_o(E_i)}{\Delta E_i} e^{-\mu(E_i)D}}{D \sum\limits_{i=1}^{n} \dfrac{\Delta I_o(E_i)}{\Delta E_i}} \quad \ldots \ldots \ldots \ldots \ldots (13.13)$$

In the calculation of the curves of Fig.3.1, a value of $D = 20$ cm has been chosen, and the diameter of the spherical model, $d = 2R$ used as a parameter. Thus the volume concentration , c, of the contrast medium Isopaque Coronar ® has been found by SNEEK (1971, internal report M82) as a function of the tube voltage for an admissible relative volume error of 1%, for different values of the diameter.

The relevant curves have been shown as Fig. 3.1 in section III.2.

['] Courtesy of Philips Medical Systems Division, Physical-technical laboratory; private communication of F. Timmer; H. Reitsma and H. Diebels (1971).

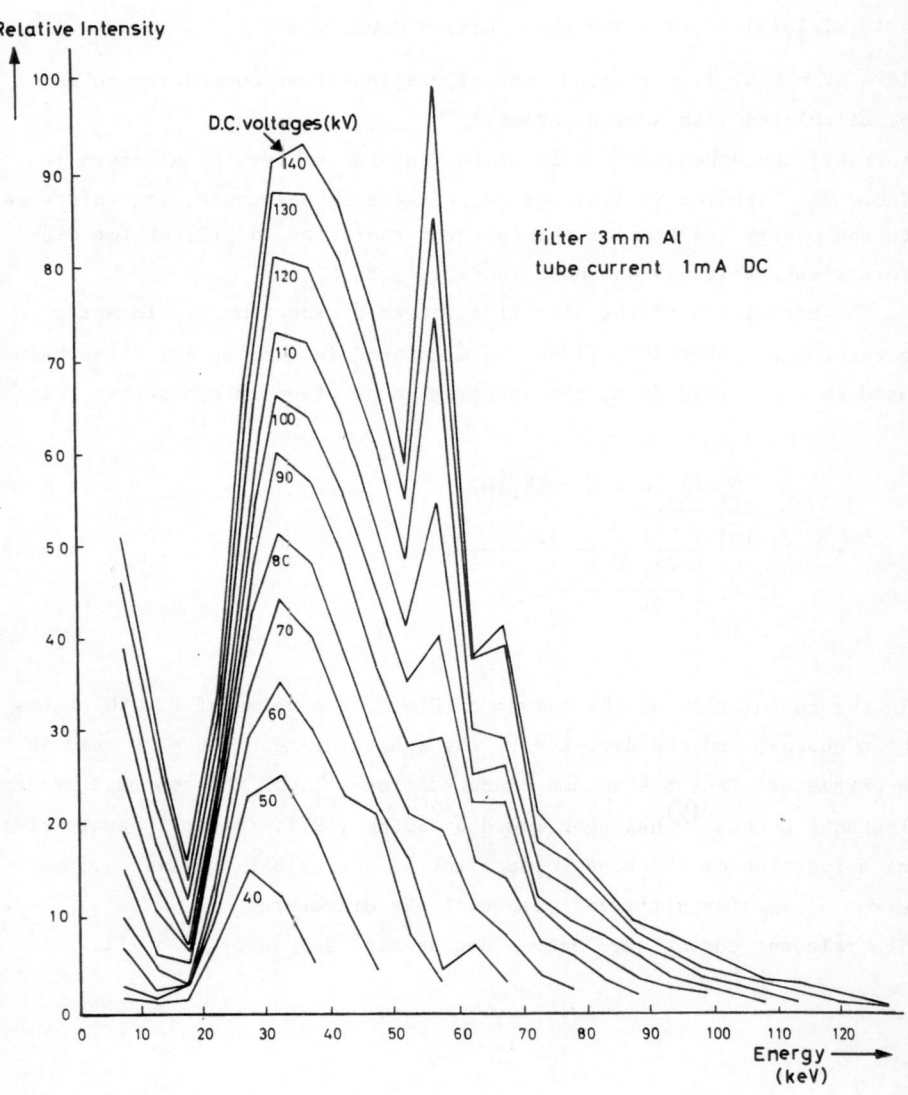

Fig. 13.2 Approximate X-ray Energy Distribution
of tubes provided with a tungsten anode

(The spectra have been reduced to a low number of histogram classes)

2.2. Correction Procedure for Low-frequency-drop in MTF

To explain the procedure according to which the edge response of an imaging system is used to correct the MTF_s for low spatial frequencies, the following derivation is given. It is a summary of the original article by TIMMER (1973).

A uni-directional MTF_s in the x-direction is defined by

$$MTF_s(\nu) = \left| \frac{\int\limits_{-\infty}^{+\infty} 1(x) \exp(-j2\pi\nu x)\, dx}{\int\limits_{-\infty}^{+\infty} 1(x)\, dx} \right| \quad\quad\quad\quad\quad (13.14)$$

in which expression $1(x)$ denotes the line-spread function (LSF).
The denominator provides a normalization, such that $MTF_s(0) = 1$. In practice, the integration limits are restricted to the diameter of the input plane of the imaging device. Moreover, if there is a foot in the LSF, the latter can only be determined in the interval $(-a, +a)$ due to noise on the base-line level of the measuring system. Using $-a$ and $+a$ as integration limits in the denominator of (13.14) instead of $-\infty$ and $+\infty$ leads to an incorrect normalization to the zero frequency. The integrated values of the truncated parts of the LSF can be estimated from the edge response

$$h(x) = C \int\limits_{-\infty}^{x} 1(u)\, du \quad\quad\quad\quad\quad\quad\quad (13.15)$$

in which expression C arises from the differences between the signal powers of the wire and edge responses. The latter rises above the noise level much more rapidly than the LSF does, say at spatial co-ordinate values $-b$ and $+b$. Here, it must be assumed that $1(x)$ and $h(x)$ are measured with the same instrument profile, (*e.g.* number of samples per unit of length). Due to time limitations, this has not been the case in Fig. 2.5[a]. Using $-b$ and $+b$ as integration limits, the denominator of (13.14) is approximated within a few percent.

Making use of (13.15), the following expression is found

$$\int_{-\infty}^{+\infty} 1(x) \, dx \simeq \int_{-b}^{+b} 1(x) \, dx = \frac{h(b) - h(-b)}{h(a) - h(-a)} \int_{-a}^{+a} 1(x) \, dx \quad \cdot \cdot \cdot \cdot \cdot \cdot \cdot \cdot \quad (13.16)$$

Thus, the corrected MTF_s is in good approximation, $(\nu \gtreqless 1/2a)$,

$$MTF_s(\nu) \simeq \left| \frac{\int_{-a}^{+a} 1(x) \exp(-j2\pi\nu x) \, dx}{\dfrac{h(b) - h(-b)}{h(a) - h(-a)} \int_{-a}^{+a} 1(x) \, dx} \right| \quad \cdot \cdot \cdot \cdot \cdot \cdot \cdot \cdot \cdot \cdot \quad (13.17^a)$$

$$MTF_s(0) = 1 \quad \cdot \cdot \cdot \cdot \cdot \cdot \cdot \cdot \cdot \cdot \cdot \cdot \cdot \cdot \cdot \cdot \cdot \cdot \cdot \quad (13.17^b)$$

This is the result, depicted in curve B of Fig. 2.5[b].

3. Results

3.1. Table 3.2.

Linear extinction coefficients of Isopaque Coronar ®at different
quantum energies (calculated by SNEEK, internal report M82):

Quantum energy E	μ_c	$\Delta\mu = \mu_c - \mu_w$	Contribution of iodine to μ_c
(keV)	(cm^{-1})	(cm^{-1})	(cm^{-1})
20	9.66	8.85	8.92
30	5.16	4.82	4.83
40	8.43	8.18	8.18
50	5.02	4.80	4.80
60	3.10	2.90	2.90
70	2.23	2.05	2.05
80	1.59	1.41	1.41
90	1.24	1.07	1.07
100	0.950	0.782	0.781
110	0.798	0.633	0.632

From the last two columns it appears that the contrast in the X-ray
picture is mainly caused by the iodine.

3.2. Table 3.3.

Comparison of concentrations of Isopaque Coronar Ⓡ, in a cylindrical phantom at various tube voltages (according to SNEEK, internal report M82):

Cylinder diameter (cm)	X-ray tube voltage (kV)								
	50			65			80		
	A	B	C	A	B	C	A	B	C
5.0	4.8	2.0	1.8	4.8	2.0	2.3	4.8	3.8	2.7
4.5	4.8	2.9	2.0	4.8	2.0	2.5	5.7	3.8	3.0
4.0	4.8	2.9	2.2	5.7	2.0	2.8	5.7	4.8	3.3
3.5	5.7	2.9	2.5	6.5	2.0	3.2	6.5	4.8	3.8
3.0	7.4	2.9	3.0	6.5	2.9	3.7	7.4	4.8	4.4
2.5	8.3	4.8	3.6	7.4	3.8	4.4	7.4	4.8	5.3
2.0	8.3	4.8	4.5	8.3	4.8	9.1	9.1	5.7	6.7

A = concentration required for adequate visual recognition of the cylinder contour on the TV-monitor

B = minimal concentration required for a detected diameter which is 1 mm smaller than the known diameter

C = concentration as derived from Fig. 3.1.

3.3 Results of In Vivo Tests.

The following regression equations and correlation coefficients have been obtained.

a. $X = EDV_{vWvB}$; $Y_1 = EDV_{Chap.}$; $Y_2 = EDV_{Dodge}$:

Dog 1:	$Y_1 = 0.97X + 1.28$	;	r=0.995	; n=10 ;	$Y_2 = 1.06X + 0.70$	;	r=0.999	; n=10
2:	1.02	0.57	0.993	13	1.08	0.26	0.999	13
3:	1.04	0.62	0.996	11	1.09	0.64	0.993	11
4:	1.09	0.06	0.999	20	1.13	0.03	1.	20
Total :	1.11	- 0.35	0.992	54	1.18	- 0.76	0.992	54

b. $X = ESV_{vWvB}$; $Y_1 = ESV_{Chap.}$; $Y_2 = ESV_{Dodge}$:

Dog 1:	$Y_1 = 0.95X + 0.64$	;	r=0.997	; n=10 ;	$Y_2 = 1.05X + 0.37$	;	r=0.999	; n=10
2:	1.08	- 0.08	1.	13	1.11	- 0.03	1.	13
3:	0.93	0.97	0.978	11	0.82	1.73	0.965	11
4:	1.08	0.16	0.990	20	1.13	0.13	0.996	20
Total :	0.98	0.56	0.984	54	1.04	0.50	0.988	54

c. $X = SV_{vWvB}$; $Y = SV_{EM}$:

Dog 1:	$Y = 0.93X + 0.27$	;	r=0.970	; n=10 ;	$X = 1.02Y + 0.16$	;	r=0.970	; n=10
2:	0.09	5.22	0.118	13	0.16	5.65	0.118	13
3:	0.31	5.26	0.639	11	1.33	- 2.36	0.639	11
4:	0.62	3.51	0.626	20	0.64	3.04	0.626	20
Total :	0.92	0.47	0.813	54	0.72	2.28	0.813	54

d. 95% confidence limits (for totals only):

Regression equation: $Y = bX + a$; $X = EDV_{vWvB}$ resp. ESV_{vWvB}

$EDV_{Chap.}$: $-0.39 < a < -0.31$; $1.07 < b < 1.15$; EDV_{Dodge}: $-0.81 < a < -0.71$; $1.13 < b < 1.23$

$ESV_{Chap.}$: $0.52 < a < 0.60$; $0.92 < b < 1.04$; ESV_{Dodge}: $0.47 < a < 0.54$; $0.99 < b < 1.09$

SV: Correlation coefficient: $0.7 < \rho < 0.9$

3.4. Results of Uncertainty Analysis

Table 11.1

i	Relevant Variables Uncertainty Interval Description	v_i w_i	Sensit. $\frac{\partial R}{\partial v_i}$	Propagation $\left\| \frac{\partial R}{\partial v_i} \cdot w_i \right\|$	$\left(\frac{\partial R}{\partial v_i} \cdot w_i \right)^2$
1	Focus-obj. distance,lat.,(D_1) (mm)	$2.0\ 10^0$	$4.20\ 10^{-3}$	$8.40\ 10^{-3}$	$7.06\ 10^{-5}$
2	Object-II. distance,lat.,(D_2) (mm)	$2.0\ 10^0$	$-9.70\ 10^{-3}$	$1.94\ 10^{-2}$	$3.76\ 10^{-4}$
3	Focus-obj. distance,front.,(L_1) (mm)	$2.0\ 10^0$	$5.40\ 10^{-3}$	$1.08\ 10^{-2}$	$1.17\ 10^{-4}$
4	Object-II. distance,front.,(L_2) (mm)	$2.0\ 10^0$	$-8.10\ 10^{-3}$	$1.62\ 10^{-2}$	$2.62\ 10^{-4}$
5	Axis slope in lat. proj. (deg)	$2.1\ 10^0$	$1.36\ 10^{-2}$	$2.86\ 10^{-2}$	$8.18\ 10^{-4}$
6	Axis ordinate intercept (lat.) (mm)	$3.0\ 10^0$	$7.20\ 10^{-3}$	$2.16\ 10^{-2}$	$4.67\ 10^{-4}$
7	Axis slope in front. proj. (deg)	$2.1\ 10^0$	$1.73\ 10^{-2}$	$3.63\ 10^{-2}$	$1.32\ 10^{-3}$
8	Axis ordinate intercept (front.) (mm)	$3.0\ 10^0$	$1.20\ 10^{-2}$	$3.60\ 10^{-2}$	$1.30\ 10^{-3}$
9	Axis length (lat. proj.) (mm)	$6.0\ 10^0$	$4.30\ 10^{-3}$	$2.58\ 10^{-2}$	$6.66\ 10^{-4}$
10	Axis length (lat. proj.) (mm)	$3.0\ 10^0$	$5.20\ 10^{-3}$	$1.56\ 10^{-2}$	$2.43\ 10^{-4}$
11	$(\bar{x}_i)_1$ ⎫ Means in three (mm)	$3.0\ 10^0$	$4.36\ 10^{-2}$	$1.31\ 10^{-1}$	$1.72\ 10^{-2}$
12	$(\bar{x}_i)_2$ ⎬ equal groups of (mm)	$3.0\ 10^0$	$5.18\ 10^{-2}$	$1.55\ 10^{-1}$	$2.40\ 10^{-2}$
13	$(\bar{x}_i)_3$ ⎭ lat. diameters (ES) (mm)	$3.0\ 10^0$	$1.21\ 10^{-2}$	$3.63\ 10^{-2}$	$1.32\ 10^{-3}$
14	$(\bar{y}_i)_1$ ⎫ Means in three (mm)	$3.0\ 10^0$	$3.80\ 10^{-2}$	$1.14\ 10^{-1}$	$1.30\ 10^{-2}$
15	$(\bar{y}_i)_2$ ⎬ equal groups of (mm)	$3.0\ 10^0$	$4.25\ 10^{-2}$	$1.28\ 10^{-1}$	$1.64\ 10^{-2}$
16	$(\bar{y}_i)_3$ ⎭ front. diameters (ES) (mm)	$3.0\ 10^0$	$1.31\ 10^{-2}$	$3.93\ 10^{-2}$	$1.54\ 10^{-3}$
17	$(\bar{\alpha}_i)_1$ ⎫	$1.0\ 10^{-1}$	$8.81\ 10^{-1}$	$8.81\ 10^{-2}$	$7.76\ 10^{-3}$
18	$(\bar{\alpha}_i)_2$ Means in six equal groups	$7.0\ 10^{-2}$	$1.97\ 10^0$	$1.38\ 10^{-1}$	$1.90\ 10^{-2}$
19	$(\bar{\alpha}_i)_3$ of indices of irregularity	$4.5\ 10^{-2}$	$2.56\ 10^0$	$1.15\ 10^{-1}$	$1.32\ 10^{-2}$
20	$(\bar{\alpha}_i)_4$ (ES) (dimensionless)	$4.0\ 10^{-2}$	$2.63\ 10^0$	$1.05\ 10^{-1}$	$1.10\ 10^{-2}$
21	$(\bar{\alpha}_i)_5$ ⎬	$6.0\ 10^{-2}$	$8.07\ 10^{-1}$	$4.84\ 10^{-2}$	$2.34\ 10^{-3}$
22	$(\bar{\alpha}_i)_6$ ⎭	$6.0\ 10^{-2}$	$3.42\ 10^{-1}$	$2.05\ 10^{-2}$	$4.20\ 10^{-4}$

Total: $1.34\ 10^0$; $1.33\ 10^{-1}$

========= =========

XIV. <u>REFERENCES</u>

1. Literature

ALDERMAN,E.L.;SANDLER,H.;BROOKER,J.Z.;SANDERS,W.J.;SIMPSON,C. and HARRISON,D.C.:
   Light-pen computer processing of video image for the determination of left
   ventricular volume. Circulation,$\underline{47}$,1973,309.
ANSELL,G.: Adverse reactions to contrast agents. Invest.Radiol.$\underline{5}$,1970,374.
ARDRAN,G.M.;HAMILL,J.;EMRYS-ROBERTS,E. and OLIVER,R.: Radiation dose to the pa-
   tient in cardiac radiology. Brit.J.Radiol.$\underline{43}$,1970,391.
ARVIDSSON,H. and OEDMAN,P.: Angiocardiography in mitral disease. Acta Radiol.
   Stockholm,$\underline{47}$,1957,97.
ARVIDSSON,H.: Angiocardiographic determination of left ventricular volume. Acta
   Radiol. Stockholm,$\underline{56}$,1961,321.
ARVIDSSON,H.: Angiocardiographic measurements in congenital heart disease (III).
   Acta Radiol. Diagn.$\underline{4}$,1966,155.
ARVIDSSON,H.: Angiocardiographic determination of left ventricular volume and
   its applications. Radiologe,$\underline{7}$,1967,200.
BAILY,N.A. and CREPEAU,R.L.: Capabilities of a single scan TV-radiographic system
   for digital data acquisition. Invest,Radiol.$\underline{6}$,1971,273.
BAKER,L.R.: Status of optical transfer function in 1970. In: Proc.Electro-
   optical Systems Design Conference, New York City,22-24 sep.1970,801.
BAKER,O.;KHALAF,J. and CHAPMAN.C.B.: A scanner-computer for determining the vo-
   lumes of cardiac chambers from cinefluorographic films. Amer.Heart J.$\underline{62}$,1961,
   797.
BAKER,V.D. and MILLER,W.B.: A TV-system for electronic radiography. In: Proc.20th.
   Ann.Conf. on Engng. in Med. and Biol. Boston,13-16 Nov.1967,Sess.10.1.
BARDEEN,C.R.: Determination of the size of the heart by means of X-rays. Amer.J.
   Anat.$\underline{23}$,1918,423.
BARNARD,A.C.L.;DUCK,I.M.;LYNN,M.S. and TIMLAKE,W.P.: The application of electro-
   magnetic theory to electrocardiology. Biophys.J.$\underline{7}$,1967,463.
BARON,M.G.: Angiocardiographic determination of ejection fractions in coronary
   artery disease. Amer.J.Cardiol.$\underline{31}$,1973,803.
BARRY,W.F.;MACINTOSH,H.D. and WHALEN,R.E.: Image distortion in cineradiographic
   equipment. Radiology,$\underline{81}$,1963,508.
BAUEREISEN,E;HAUCK,G.;JACOB,R. und PEIPER,U.: Enddiastolische Druck-volumen Re-
   lationen und Arbeitsdiagramme des intakten Herzens im natürlichen Kreislauf
   in Abhängigkeit von Herzfrequenz, Adrenalinwirkung und Vagusreiz. Pflügers
   Arch.Ges.Physiol.$\underline{281}$,1964,216.

BECKENBACH,E.S.: Some aspects of the computerization of high-speed cineangiographic left ventricular volume determination. Thesis,U.C.L.A.,1969.

BENTIVOGLIO,L.G.;GRIFFITH,L.D.;CUESTA,A.J. and GECZY,M.: Radiographic evaluation
of formulas for left ventricular volume using canine casts. J.Appl.Physiol.
33,1972,365.

BERGSTROM,K.;ERIKSON,U. and GUSTAFSSON,B.: Roentgenological heart volume determination. Acta Soc.Med.Upsalien.74,1969(a),49;74,1969(b),81.

BESSE,P.;LEGOFF,G.;CHARLAND,R.;LE FRANC,G et BRICAUD,H.: Evaluation angiographique quantitative des volumes de la cinétique ventriculaire gauche: Etude
critique. Arch.Mal.Coeur,67,1974,1075.

BIBERMAN,L.M.: Perception of displayed information. Editor:L.M.Biberman. New York
1973.

BISCHOFF,K.: Die Bedeutung des Röntgenfernsehens für die Erweiterung des Durch-
leuchteinsatzes in der medizinischen Diagnostik. Fortschr.Röntgenstr.95,1961,
104.

BISCHOFF,K.: Der Wert der Strahlenpulsung bei den modernen Verfahren der Röntgen
Kinematographie. Fortschr.Röntgenstr.97,1962,82.

BJOERK,L.: Semi-automatic construction and computer analysis of volume curves
and pressure-volume curves in left ventricular cineangiography. Acta Radiol.
Diagn.10,1970,413.

BLINKS,J.R. and KOCK-WESER,J.: Physical factors in the analysis of the actions
of drugs on myocardial contractility. Pharmacol.Rev.15,1963,531.

BLUM,H.: A transformation for extracting new descriptors of shape. In: Models
for the perception of speech and visual form. Editor: W. Wathen-Dunn.
Cambridge,1964,362.

BOM,N.: New concepts in echocardiography. Thesis, Rotterdam,1972.

BOOM,H.B.K.;DENIER VAN DER GON,J.J.;NIEUWENHUYS,J.H.M. and SCHIERECK,P.: Cardiac
contractility. Actin-myosin interaction as measured from the left ventricular
pressure curve. Europ.J.Cardiol.1,1974,217.

BOOTSMA,B.K.;HOELEN,A.J.;STRACKEE,J. and MEIJLER,F.L.: Analysis of RR-intervals
in patients with atrial fibrillation at rest and during exercise. Circulation,
41,1970,783.

BORGMAN,N.J.: Electronic scanning for variable stars. Thesis, Groningen,1956.

BOUWERS,A.: Der Informationseinhalt des Röntgenbildes. Röntgen-Bl.15,1962,81.

BOVE,A.A. and GIMENEZ,J.L.: Computer analysis of flow characteristics of injection catheters. Invest.Radiol.3,1968,427.

BOVE,A.A.: A cineradiographic study of left ventricular physiology in the dog.
Thesis, Phiadelphia,1970(a).

BOVE,A.A. and LYNCH,P.R.: Measurement of canine left ventricular performance by
cineradiography of the heart. J.Appl.Physiol.29,1970(b),877.

BOVE,A.A.;ZISKIN,M.C.;FREEMAN,E.;GIMENEZ,J.L. and LYNCH,P.R.: Selection of opti-
mum cineradiographic frame rate, relation to accuracy of cardiac measurements.
Invest.Radiol.5,1970(c),329

BRAUN,H.: Das Herzvolumen und seine Beziehung zu den anderen hämodynamischen
Faktoren unter Anwendung neuer Röntgenologischer Untersuchungsmethoden. Arch.
Kreisl.Forsch.32,1960,87.

BRAUNWALD,E.;ROSS,J. and SONNENBLICK,E.H.: Mechanics of concentration in the normal and failing heart. New Engl.J.Med. Medical Progress Series, London,1967.

BRISTOW,J.D.;FERGUSON,R.E.;MINTZ,F. and RAPAPORT,E.: The influence of heart rate
on left ventricular volume in dogs. J.Clin.Invest.42,1963,649.

BROUSTET,P.;WANGERMEZ,CH. et GUILLON,P.: Mesure du volume cardiaque par la tomographie axiale. Arch.Mal.Coeur,46,1953,143.

BROUSTET,P.;WANGERMEZ,CH.;MARTIN,P.L.;DUHAMEL,J. et BRICAUD,H.: Etude du volume
cardiaque par la tomographie axiale transverse. J.Radiol.Electrol.36,1955,770.

BROUSTET,P.;WANGERMEZ,CH.;DUHAMEL,J.;MARTIN,P.L.;BRICAUD,H. et FONTANILLE,P.:
Etude comparative des resultats des mesures du volume cardiaque par la méthode
de stratigraphie axiale transverse et les méthodes géometriques téléradio-
graphiques. J.Radiol.Electrol.41,1960,417.

186

BROUSTET,P.;WANGERMEZ,CH. et BRICAUD,H.: Mesure du volume du coeur pathologique. Arch.Mal.Coeur,54,1961,877.

BRUN,P.;GESCHWIND,H,;HERREMAN,F. et CAMPAGNAC,J.: Etude de l'activité méchanique du ventricule gauche par calcul sur ordinateur à partir des données cinéangiographiques et hémodynamiques. Arch.Ma.Coeur,61,1968,135.

BRUN,P.;NIAY,E. et SEGELLE,R.: Système informatique pour la mesure des volumes cardiaques par cinéangiographie biplane rapide. Onde Electrique,50,1970,395.

BRUN,P.;CANNET,G. et HERREMAN,F.: La mesure du volume endocavitaire ventriculaire gauche par méthode angiographique. Acta Cardiol. (Brux.),27,1972,271.

BRUTSAERT,D.L. and SONNENBLICK,E.H.: Force-velocity-length-time relations of the contractile elements in heart muscle of the cat. Circulat.Res.24,1969,137.

BRUTSAERT,D.L. and SONNENBLICK,E.H.: Cardiac muscle mechanics in the evaluation of myocardial contractility and pump function: problems, concepts and directions. Progr.Cardiovasc.Dis.16,1973,337.

BUECHNER,H.: Telediametry: the reading of absolute measures from the TV-screen in image intensifier TV-fluoroscopy. Fortschr.Röntgenstr.109,1968,226.

BUERSCH,J.: Quantitative Videodensitometrie. Habil.Schrift, Kiel,1972.

BUGGE,J.: A standardized plastic injection technique for anatomical purposes. Acta Anat.54,1963,177.

BUNNELL,I.L.;GRANT,C. and.GREENE,D.G.: Left ventricular function derived from the pressure-volume diagram. Amer.J.Med.39,1965,881.

CALVERT,M.H. and HEATON,A.G.: Stroke volume measurement in animals with pacemaker control of heart rate. Cardiovasc.Res.7,1973,719.

CARLETON,R.A.: Change in left ventricular volume during angiocardiography. Amer. J.Cardiol.27,1971,460.

CARLSSON,E and LOVE,J.W.: Lead coating of the tricuspid valve in dogs. Acta Radiol.Diagn.2,1964,517.

CARLSSON,E.: Angiocardiographic measurements of the cardiac ventricles in dogs. Acta Radiol.Diagn.4,1966,671.

CARLSSON,E. and MILNE,E.N.C.: Permanent implantation of endocardial tantalum screws: A new technique for functional studies of the heart in the experimental animal. J.Canad.Ass.Radiol.19,1967,304.

CARLSSON,E.: Experimental studies of ventricular mechanics in dogs using tantalum labeled heart. Fed.Proc.28,1969,1324.

CARLSSON,E.: Measurement of cardiac chamber volumes and dimensions by radiographic methods. Thesis, Berkeley,1970.

CHAMBERLAIN,W.E. and DOCK,W.: The study of the heart with the röntgen-cinematograph. Radiology,7,1926,185.

CHANG,S.K.: The reconstruction of binary patterns from their projections. Commun. Ass.Comput.Mach.14,1971(a),21.

CHANG,S.K. and SHELTON,G.L.: Two alorithms for multiple-view binary pattern reconstruction. IEEE Trans.SMC.1,1971(b),90.

CHANG,S.K. and CHOW,C.K.: The reconstruction of three-dimensional objects from two orthogonal projections and its application to cardiac cineangiography. IEEE Trans.C.22,1973,18.

CHAPMAN,C.B.;BAKER,O.;REYNOLDS,J. and BONTE,F.: Use of biplane cinefluorography for measurement of ventricular volume. Circulation,18,1958,1105.

CHAPMAN,C.B.;BAKER,O.;MITCHELL,J.H. and COLLIER,R.G.: Experiences with a cinefluorographic method for measuring ventricular volume. Amer.J.Cardiol.18,1966, 25.

CHEN,J.T.T.;MACINTOSH,H.D.;CAPP,M.P.;MORRIS,J.J.;CANENT,R.V. and LESTER,R.G.: Intercalative angiocardiography: A method for recording cardiovascular dynamics on a single film. Radiology,93,1969,499.

CHOW,C.K. and KANEKO,T.: Boundary detection of radiographic images by threshold method. Report RC3203 (14528)IBM, Thomas J.Watson Res.Center, Yorktown Heights 1970.

CHOW,C.K. and KANEKO,T.: Computer calculation of left ventricular volumes from a cineangiogram. In: Proc.S.P.I.E. Seminar Quant.Imaginary in the Bio-Med. Sciences. Editor: R.E. Herron, Houston,10-12 May 1971,251.

CHOW,C.K. and KANEKO,T.: Automatic boundary detection of the left ventricle from cineangiograms. Comput.Biomed.Res.5,1972,388.

CHOW,C.K.;HILAL,S.K. and NIEBUHR,K.E.: X-ray image subtraction by digital means. IBM J.Res.Develop.17,1973,206.

CLARKE,H.C.: A contouring device for use in radiation treatment planning. Brit. J.Radiol.42,1969,858.

CLAYTON,P.D.;HARRIS,L.D.;RUMEL,S.R. and WARNER,H.R.: Left ventricular videometry. Comput.Biomed.Res.7,1974,369.

COLTMAN,J.W.: Fluoroscopic image brightening by electronic means. Radiology,51, 1947,359.

COULAM,C.M.;GREENLEAF,J.F.;TSAKIRIS,A.G. and WOOD,E.H.: Three-dimensional computerized display of physiologic models and data. Comput.Biomed.Res.5,1972,166.

COVVEY,J.D.;ADELMAN,A.G.;FELDERHOF,C.H.;MENDLER,P;WIGLE,E.D. and TAYLOR,K.W.: The television/computer system-the acquisition and processing of cardiac catheterization data using a small computer. In: Proc.A.F.I.P.S. Fall Joint Computer Conference,39,1971(a),455.

COVVEY,H.D.;HALL,W.: Television as a computer peripheral. In: Proc.Decus Meeting, 1971(b),63.

COVVEY,H.D.;ADELMAN,A.G.;FELDERHOF,C.H.;TAYLOR,K.W. and WISE,E.D.: Television/computerdimensional analysis interface with special application to left ventricular cineangiograms. Comput. Biol.Med.2,1972,221.

CRAIGE,E,;FORTUIN,N.J.;SHERMAN,M.E. and HOOD,W.P.: Determination of left ventricular volume and ejection fraction by echocardiography. In: Quantitation in cardiology. Editors: H.A. Snellen,H.C. Hemker,P.G. Hugenholtz and J.H. van Bemmel. Leiden,1972,204.

CRITTENDEN,J.J. and STERN,C.A.: Simplified subtraction. Amer.J.Roentgenol.97, 1966,523.

CROWTHER,D.A.;ROSIER,D.J.DE and KLUG,A.: The reconstruction of a three-dimensional structure from projections and its application to electron microscopy. Proc.Roy,Soc.,Ser.A,317,1970(a),319.

CROWTHER,R.A.;AMOS,L.A.;FINCH,J.T.;ROSIER,D.J.DE and KLUG,A.: Three-dimensional reconstruction of spherical viruses by Fourier synthesis from electron micrographs. Nature,226,1970(b),421.

CSORBA,I.P.: Contrast characteristics of X-ray images. R.C.A.Rev.32,1971,150.

DAHLSTROEM,K.: Ca-Mg-balanced Isopaque-A low-viscosity preparation. Acta Radiol. Supp.270,1966,143.

DAUGHTERS,G.T.;INGELS,N.B.;CARRERA,C.J.;WEXTER,L. and SMITH,N.T.: Regional myocardial dynamics from single plane coronary cineangiograms. J.Biomech.6,1973, 25.

DAVIDSE,J.;JONG,L.P.DE and SLAGER,C.J.: Automatic detection of the left ventricular outline in angiograms using television signal processing techniques. In: Dig.Europ.Conf.Electronics 'Eurocon'74', Amsterdam,22-26 April 1974, Sess. E-4-4.

DAVILA,J.C.: Introduction to symposium on measurement of left ventricular volume. Amer.J.Cardiol.18,1966(a),1.

DAVILA,J.C. and SANMARCO,M.E.: An analysis of the fit of mathematical models applicable to the measurement of left ventricular volume. Amer.J.Cardiol.18, 1966(b),31.

DEAN,R.R.: The physiologic and toxic consequences of the intracoronary administration of certain radiopaque contrast agents. Thesis,Michigan,1966.

DESILETS,D.F. and BECKENBACH,E.S.: Myocardial function from cineangiograms with a digital computer. Radiology,39,1971,319.

DIEREN,A.VAN en WIJKMANS,D.W.: Vacuum vormfixatie op de operatietafel. Biotechniek,12,1973,117.

DINN,D.I.;WINTER,D.A. and TRENHOLM,B.G.: CINTEL, computer interface for television. IEEE Trans.C-19,1970,1091.

DODGE,H.T. and TANENBAUM,H.L.: Left ventricular volume in normal man and alterations with disease. Circulation,14,1956,927.

DODGE,H.T.;SANDLER,H.;BALLEW,D.H. and LORD,J.D.: The use of biplane angio cardio-
graphy for the measurement of left ventricular volume in man. Amer.Heart J.60,
1960,762.
DODGE,H.T.;HAY,R.E. and SANDLER,H.: Pressure-volume characteristics of the dias-
tolic left ventricle of man with heart disease. Amer.Heart J.64,1962,503.
DODGE,H.T.;SANDLER,H.;BAXLEY,W.A. and HAWLEY,R.R.: Usefullness and limitations
of radiographic methods for determining left ventricular volume. Amer.J.
Cardiol.18,1966,10.
DODGE,H.T.: Measurement of heart chamber volumes and dimensions, introduction.
In: Proc. Summer Workshop Council on Basic Science, Amer.Heart Assn. Denver,
24-27 Juli 1967,1.
DONATO,L.;GIUNTINI,C. and LEWIS,M.L.: Quantitative radiocardiography (I and II).
Circulation,26,1962(a),174 and Circulation,26,1962(b),183.
DORPH,S.;MYGIND,T.;NORTHEVED,A.;OKHOLM,B.;PETERSEN,O. and OIGAARD,A.: A dose-
reducing fluoroscopy system. Radiology,97,1970,399.
DUBOIS,E.F.: Basal metabolism in health and disease,1927. (Quoted in: Jonsell,
1939).
DUEMMLING,K.: Verminderung störender Trägheitseffekte bei der Stereodurch-
leuchtung und bei der Stereo- und Hochfrequenzkinematographie. Röntgenpraxis,
22,1969(a),271.
DUEMMLING,K.: Bildgütetest für Bildverstärker- und Fernsehanlagen. Röntgenpraxis,
22,1969(b),190.
DUEMMLING,K.: Bewegungsregistrierung mit Röntgenbildverstärker- Kino- und Fernsehanlagen. Biomediz.Techn.17,1972,203.
DUHAMEL,I.;MARTIN,P.I.;GUILLON,M. et BROUSSIN,S.: La méthode tomographique dans
la mesure du volume d'un viscère plein. Application au coeur. Acta Radiol.41,
1954,377.
DIJKEMA,F.K. and ELZINGA,G.: Integrator for aortic and pulmonary artery flow
signals, with automatic zero adjustment and beat-to-beat mean flow computation
Cardiovasc.7,1973,572.
EPHRAIM,K.H. (Chairman): Report preliminary working-group "Standaardisering me-
thoden en technieken medische informatieverwerking." V.M.B.I.-Meded.3,1974,1.
ETT,A.H. and MERRITT,E.W.: 4481 Film reader/recorder, basic system operation.
I.B.M.Comm.Engng.Sci.Cent.1971,1.
EVANS,D.W. and CARPENTER,P.B.: Errors involved in radiological heart volume de-
termination by the ellipsoid-approximation technique. Brit.Heart J.27,1965,429
EYKMAN,P.H.: Roentgen-cinematography. Arch.Roentgen-Ray,13,1909,261.
FEDDEMA,J. and BOTDEN,P.J.M.: Adequate diagnostic information. In: Television in
diagnostic radiology. Editors: R.D. Moseley and J.H. Rust, Birmingham,1969,15.
FISCHER,V.J.;LEE,R.J. and KAVALER,F.: The heterogeneous contractile performance
of the left ventricle. In: Factors influencing myocardial contractility.
Editors R.D. Tanz,F. Kavaler and J. Roberts, New York,1967,113.
FONTANILLE,P.: La mesure du volume cardiaque en pathologie par les méthodes
radiologiques. Thesis,Bordeaux,1960,217.
FOX,I.J. and WOOD,E.H.: Symposium in indocyanine green and its applications.
Mayo Clinic Proc.37,1960,729.
FRANK,O.: Zur Dynamik des Herzmuskels. Z.Biol.32,1895,370.
FRANKEN,A.A. and SCHEREN,W.J.L.: The influence of the camera tube on the temporal
modulation transfer function in diagnostic X-ray television. Medica Mundi,17,
1972,121.
FREEMAN,E.: On the encoding of arbitrary geometric configurations. IRE Trans.
Elec.Comp.Ec-10,1961,260.
FREEMAN,E.;ZISKIN,M.C.;BOVE,A.A.;GIMINEZ,J.L. and LYNCH,P.R.: Cineradiographic
frame rate selection for left ventricular volumetry. Radiology,96,1970,587.
FRIEDELL,H.L. and GREGG,E.C.: Radiologic and allied procedures from the point of
view of information content and visual perception. Amer.J.Radiol.94,1965,719.
FRIEDER,G. and HERMAN,G.T.: Resolution in reconstructing objects from electron
micrographs. J.Theor.Biol.33,1971,189.

FROESCHLE,E,;SOTTA,H. and RACKETTE,K.H.: Recording with a TV-camera into the PDP-
8's core memory. In: Proc.Decus Meeting,1971,169.
GAUER,O.H.: Volume changes of the left ventricle during blood pooling and exer-
cise in the intact animal: their effect on left ventricular performance.
Physiol.Rev.35,1955,143.
GEBAUER,A.;LISSNER,J. und SCHOTT,O.: Das Röntgenfernsehen. Technische Grundlagen
und klinisch-röntgenologische Anwendung. Stuttgart,1965.
GEBHARDT,W.: Eine neue Methode der röntgenologischen Herzvolumenbestimmung mit
Hilfe des simultanen Schichtverfahrens in Vergleich mit den bisher üblichen
Methoden. Klin.Wochenschr.35,1957,1119.
GEBHARDT,W.;DANNER,D.;REINDELL,H. und KOENIG,K.: Eine vergleichende Untersuchung
zur methodischen Fehlerbreite der röntgenologischen Herzvolumenbestimmung.
Acta Med.Scand.167,1960,467.
GEIGEL,R.: Die klinische Verwertung der Herzsilhouette. Münch.Mediz.Wochenschr.
61,1914,1220.
GHISTA,D.N. and SANDLER,H.: An analytic elestic-visco-elastic model for the
shape and the forces in the left ventricle. J.Biomech.2,1969,35.
GHISTA,D.N.;PATIL,K.M.;GOULD,P. and WOO,K.B.: Computerized left ventricular me-
chanics and control systems analysis models relevant for cardiac diagnosis.
Comput.Biol.Med.3,1973,27.
GLANCY,D.L. and MARCUS,M.L.: Introduction to the symposium on the use of video
technology in cardiovascular research. Amer.J.Cardiol.32,1973,135.
GOERKE,R.J. and CARLSSON,E.: Calculation of right and left cardiac ventricular
volumes.-Method using standard computer equipment and biplane angiocardio-
grams. Invest.Radiol.2,1967,360.
GOODMAN,J.W.: Introduction to Fourier Optics. New York,1968.
GOOTMAN,N.;RUDOLPH,A.M. and BUCKLEY,N.M.: Effects of angiographic contrast media
on cardiac function. Amer.J.Cardiol.25,1970,59.
GORDON,R. and HERMAN,G.T.: Reconstruction of pictures from their projections.
Commun.Ass.Comput.Mach.14,1971,759.
GOTT,A.H.;JANZ,R.F. and STIMSON,M.J.: Two-dimensional computer graphics applied
to muscle physiology. In: Quantitative imagery in the Biomedical Sciences,
Proc.S.P.I.E. Seminar-in-depth, Houston,1971,239.
GREENE,D.G.;CARLISLE,R.;GRANT,C. and BUNNELL,I.L.: Estimation of left ventricu-
lar volume by one-plane cineangiography. Circulation,35,1967,61.
GREENLEAF,J.F.;RITMAN,E.L.;COULAM,C.M.;STURM,R.E. and WOOD,E.H.: Computer graphic
techniques for study of temporal and spatial relationships of multidimensional
data derived from biplane roentgen videograms with particular reference to
cardioangiography. Comput.Biomed.Res.5,1972(a),368.
GREENLEAF,J.F.;RITMAN,E.L.;WOOD,E.H.;FRYE,R.L.;ROBB,R.A. and JOHNSON,S.A.:
Dynamic computer generated display for study of the human ventricle. In: Proc.
S.P.I.E.Seminar Developments in Electronic Imaging Techniques, San Mateo,1972
(b),32,111.
GREGG,E.C.: Assessment of radiologic imaging. Amer.J.Roentgenol.97,1966,776.
GRIBBE,P.;LIND,J.;LINKO,E. and WEGELIUS,C.: The events of the left side of the
normal heart as studied by cineradiography. Cardiologia,33,1958,293.
GRIBBE,P.;HIRVONEN,L.;LIND,J. and WEGELIUS,C.: Cineangiocardiographic recordings
of the cycle changes in volume of the left ventricle. Cardiologia,34,1959,348.
GRIBBE,P.: Comparison of the angiocardiographic and direct fick methods in determining cardiac output. Cardiologia,36,1960,20.
GRIFFITH,R.L.;GRANT,C. and KAUFMAN,H.: An algorithm for locating the aortic value
and the apex in left-ventricular angiocardiograms. IEEE Trans.Biomed.Eng.BME-
21,1974,345.
GROEDEL,F.M.: Technik der Röntgencinematographie. Deutsche Mediz.Wochenschr.35,
1909,434.
GROH,F.: Ein elektronisches Subtraktionsgerät. Röntgenpraxis,20,1967,43.
GROH,G.;KLOTZ,E. and WEISS,H.: Simple and fast method for the presentation of
the two-dimensional modulation transfer function of X-ray systems. Applied
Optics,12,1973,1693.

GROLLMAN,J.H.;KLOSTERMAN,H.;HERMAN,H.W.;MOLER,C.L.;EBER,L.M. and MACALPIN,R.N.:
   Dose reduction low pulse-rate fluoroscopy. Radiology,105,1972,293.
HAAS,C. and KUNDEL,H.L.: Television roentgen image subtraction using one camera.
   Radiology,92,1969,1118.
HALES,S.: Statical essays: containing haemastatics; or, an account of some
   hydraulick and hydrostatical experiments made on the blood and blood-vessels
   of animals. London, 1733,17.
HALL,P.: Information science, the patient and the medical practice. In: Informa-
   tion processing of medical records. Editors: J. Anderson and J.M. Forsyte,
   Amsterdam,1970,31.
HALLERMAN,F.J.;RASTELLI,G.C. and SWAN,H.J.C.: Effects of rapid injection of he-
   parinized blood into right and left ventricles of dogs. Radiology,83,1964,647.
HALLERMAN,F.J.: Leftventricular volumes in dogs measured by an indicator dilution
   and an angiographic method. Thesis, Minnesota,1965.
HAMNER,A.P. and BJOERK,L.: Measurement of left ventricular size using cineradio-
   graphic technics in one plane. Texas Rep.Biol.Med.27,1969,57.
HARRISON,D.C.;GOLDBLATT,A. and BRAUNWALD,E.: Studies on cardiac dimensions in
   intact, unanesthetized man. Circul.Res.13,1963,448.
HAWTHORNE,E.W.: Introduction to: contractile behaviour of the heart. In: Factors
   influencing myocardial contractility. Editors: R.D. Tanz;F. Kavaler and
   J. Roberts. New York,1967,137.
HAWTHORNE,E.W.: Introduction to the physiology society symposium on dynamic geo-
   metry of the left ventricle. Fed.Proc.28,1969,1323.
HEETHAAR,R.M.: A mathematical model of A-V conduction in the rat heart. Thesis,
   Utrecht,1972.
HEIKKILA,J.;TABAKIN,B.S. and HUGENHOLTZ,P.G.: Quantification of function in nor-
   mal and infarcted regions of the left ventricle. Cardiovasc.Res.6,1972,516.
HEINTZEN,P.H. und OSYPKA,P.: Quantitative Analyse der Leuchtdichte und Strah-
   lungsimpulse an Röntgen-Bildverstärker-Kinepulsanlagen. Fortschr.Röntgenstr.
   111,1969,115.
HEINTZEN,P.H.: Roentgen-,cine- and videodensitometry. Editor: P.H. Heintzen,
   Stuttgart,1971 (a).
HEINTZEN,P.H. and PILARCZYK,J.: Videodensitometry with contoured and controlled
   windows. In: Roentgen-,cine and videodensitometry. Editor: P.H. Heintzen,
   Stuttgart,1971(b),56.
HEINTZEN,P.H.;MALERCZYK,V.;PILARCZYK,J.SCHOHL,H.H. und VOGEL,G.W.: Automatisie-
   rung der röntgenologischen Herzkammervolumenbestimmung unter Einsatz eines
   magnetischen Bildplattenspeichers. Fortschr.Röntgenstr.114,1971(c),215.
HEINTZEN,P.H.;MALERCZYK,V.;PILARCZYK,J. and SCHEEL,W.: On-line processing of the
   video-image for left ventricular volume-determination. Comput.Biomed.Res.4,
   1971(d),474.
HEINTZEN,P.H.;MALERCZYK,V. and PILARCZYK,J.: A videometric technique for automated processing of pressure-volume diagrams. Comput.Biomed.Res.4,1971(e),486.
HEINTZEN,P.H.: Usefulness and limitation of conventional X-ray equipment for
   roentgendensitometric studies. In: Roentgen-,cine- and videodensitometry.
   Editor: P.H.Heintzen, Stuttgart,1971(f),1.
HEINTZEN,P.H.: Videodensitometry with pulsed radiation. In: Roentgen-,cine- and
   videodensitometry. Editor: P.H. Heintzen, Stuttgart,1971(g),46.
HEINTZEN,P.H. and MOLDENHAUER,K.: The X-ray absorption by contrast material,
   theoretical considerations. In: Roentgen-,cine- and videodensitometry. Editor:
   P.H. Heintzen, Stuttgart,1971(h),73.
HEINTZEN,P.H. and MOLDENHAUER,K.: X-ray absorption by contrast material using
   pulsed radiation. In: Roentgen-,cine- and videodensitometry. Editor:
   P.H. Heintzen, Stuttgart,1971(i),85.
HEINTZEN,P.H.;LANGE,P.E.;MALERCZYK,V.;and PILARCZYK,J.: Methods for the analysis
   of angiocardiographic data. In: Quantitation in cardiology. Editors:
   H.A. Snellen;H.C. Hemker;P.G. Hugenholtz and J.H. van Bemmel, Leiden,1972,179.

HEINTZEN,P.H.;MALERCZYK,V. und PILARCZYK,J.: Neue Verfahren zur Videodensitometrie und Videometrie. In: Densitometrie in der Radiologie. Editor: F. Heuck,
Stuttgart,1973,25.

HEINTZEN,P.H.;MOLDENHAUER,K. and LANGE,P.E.: Three-dimensional computerized contraction pattern analysis. Europ. J.Cardiol.$\underline{1}$,1974,229.

HEINZE,H.G.;RIEMANN,H. und DUEMMLING,K.: Angiographie mit Hilfe der Fernsehsub-
traktion. In: Angiographie und ihre Fortschritte. Editor: K.E. Loose,
Stuttgart,1972,34.

HELVETIUS: Observations sur l'inégalité de capacité qui se trouve entre les
organes destinés a la circulation du sang dans le corps de l'homme et sur les
changements qui arrivent au sang en passant par le poumon. Hist.Acad.Sci.Ann.
1718/$\underline{4}$,1919,222. (Quoted in: Robin,1864).

HERMANN,$\overline{H}$.J. and BARTLE,S.H.: Left ventricular volumes by angiocardiography:
comparison of methods and simplification of techniques. Cardiovasc.Res.$\underline{2}$,1968,
404.

HERSTEL,W.: Physical limitations of vision and television in X-ray fluoroscopy.
Thesis, Leiden,1968.

HEUCK,F.: Densitometrie in der Radiologie. Editor: F. Heuck, Stuttgart,1973.

HIFFELSHEIM,E. et ROBIN,CH.: Sur le rapport de la capacité de chaque oreillette
avec celle du ventricule correspondant. J.Anat.Physiol.Norm.Path., Paris,$\underline{1}$,
1864,413.

HOLLANDER,B.A.;HILAL,S.K. and SEAMAN,W.B. Evaluation of a radiographic imaging
system with a microfocal spot X-ray tube. Radiology,$\underline{103}$,1972,667.

HOLMAN,C.B. and BULLARD,F.E.: The application of closed-circuit television in
diagnostic roentgenology. Mayo Clinic Proc.$\underline{38}$,1963,67.

HOLST,G.;BOER,J.M.DE;TEVES,M.C. and VEENEMANS,$\overline{C}$.F.: Transformation of light of
long wavelength into light of short wavelength. Physics,$\underline{1}$,1934,297.

HOLT,J.P. and ALLENSWORTH,J.: Estimation of residual volume of the right ventricle of the dog's heart. Circul.Res.$\underline{5}$,1957,323.

HONDIUS BOLDINGH,W.: Grids, to reduce scattered Z-rays in medical radiography.
Thesis, Eindhoven,1964.

HOOD,W.P.;THOMSON,W.J. and RACKLEY,C.E.: Comparison of calculations of left ventricular wall stress in man from thin-walled and thick-walled ellipsoidal
models. Circulat.Res.$\underline{24}$,1969,575.

HOOPEN,M.TEN: Ventricular response in atrial fibrillation. A model based on re-
tarded excitation. Circul.Res.$\underline{19}$,1966,911.

HOOR,F.TEN and MOOK,G.A.: Calculation of the area under an indicator dilution
curve and the mean transit time of the indicator. Proc.Kon.Ned.Acad.Wet.,
Series C,$\underline{70}$,1967,466.

HOOR,F.TEN: Bepaling van de gemiddelde bloedstroomsterkte met indicatorverdun-
nings methoden. Thesis, Groningen,1969.

HUTT,P.R.: A system of data transmission in the field blanking period of the
television signal. I.B.A.Techn.Rev.$\underline{3}$,1973,37.

INGELS,N.B.;DAUGHTERS,G.T. and DAVIES,$\overline{S}$.R.: Stereo photogrammatic studies on the
dynamic geometry of the canine left ventricular epicardium. J.Biomech.$\underline{4}$,1971,
541.

ISERI,L.T.;KAPLAN,M.A.;EVANS,M.J. and NICKEL,E.D.: Effect of concentrated contrast media during angiography on plasma volume and plasma osmolality. Amer.
Heart J.$\underline{69}$,1965,154.

JAEGER,H.: Physikalisch-technischen Grundlagen zur röntgenphotographischen Ab-
bildung von Weichteilen. Röntgen.Bl.$\underline{22}$,1969,323.

JANZ,R.F. and GRIMM,A.F.: Finite-element model for the mechanical behaviour of
the left ventricle. Circul.Res.$\underline{30}$,1972,244.

JOHNSON,S.A.;ROBB,R.A.;GREENLEAF,$\overline{J}$.F.;RITMAN,E.L.;LEE,S.L.;HERMAN,G.T.;STURM,R.E.
and WOOD,E.H.: The problem of accurate measurement of left ventricular shape
and dimensions from multiplane roentgenographic data. Europ.J.Cardiol.$\underline{1}$,1974,
241.

JONSELL,S.: Method for the determination of heart size by teleroentgenology.
Acta Radiol.$\underline{20}$,1939.325.

KAHLSTORF,A.: Uber eine orthodiagraphischen Herzvolumenbestimmung. Fortschr. Röntgenstr.45,1932,123.

KANAMORI,H. and MURASHIMA,S.: Information capacity of radiographic images for the random signal and continuous objects. Jap.J.Appl.Phys.9,1970,182.

KARLINER,J.S.;GAULT,J.H.;BOUCHARD,R.J. and HOLZER,J.: Factors influencing the ejection fraction and the mean rate of circumferential shortening during atrial fibrillation in man. Cardiovasc.Res.8,1974,18.

KASSER,I.S. and WARD KENNEDY,J.: Measurement of left ventricular volumes in man by single-plane cineangiocardiography. Invest.Radiol.4,1969,83.

KAZAMIAS,T.M. and GANDER,M.P.: Left ventricular motion disorders, functional left ventricular aneurysms; their detection by radarkymography. Amer.J.Cardiol.32,1973,151.

KIMURA,E.;YAMAGUCHI,I.;KUROKAWA,A.;HYASHI,C. and HYAKAWA,H.: Automatic estimation of heart volume by 'AMDCOX'(Automatic measurement by densitometry-computer system of X-ray picture), -a preliminary report. Dig.10th.Int.Conf.Med.Biol. Engng., Dresden,13-17 Aug.1973,Sess,31-9.

KJELLBERG,E.R.;LOENNROTH,H. and RUDHE,U.: The effect of various factors on the roentgenological determination of the cardiac volume. Acta Radiol.35,1951,413.

KLEIN,A.I. and MACPHERSON,D.: Television measurement pulse generator-mixer. Med. Biol.Engng.5,1967,267.

KLINE,S.J. and MAC CLINTOCK,F.A.: Describing uncertainties in single-sample experiments. Mech.Engng.75,1953,3.

KLOSTER,F.E.;BRISTOW,J.;PORTER,G.A.;INDUINS,M.P. and GRISWOLD,H.E.: Comparative haemodynamic effects of equiosmolar injections of angiographic contrast materials. Invest.Radiol.2,1967,353.

KOENIG,K. und BICHMAN,R.: Vergleichende Untersuchungen zur röntgenologischen Herzvolumenbestimmung in Rüken- und Bauchlage. Fortschr.Röntgenstr.107,1967,38

KONG,Y.;MORRIS,J.J. and MACINTOSH,H.D.: Assessment of regional myocardial performance from biplane coronary cineangiograms. Amer.J.Cardiol.27,1971,529.

KROVETZ,L.J.;FAIRCHILD,B.T. and HARDIN,S.: An analysis of factors determining delivery rates of liquids through cardiac catheters. Radiology,86,1966,123.

KROVETZ,L.J.;SIMON,A.L. and LEVY,R.J.: Effects of angiocardiographic contrast media on left ventricular function. John Hopkins Med.J.127,1970,127.

KRUGER,R.P.: Computer processing of radiographic images. Thesis, Columbia,1971.

KRUGER,R.P.;TOWNES,J.R,;HALL,O.L.;DWYER,S.J. and LODWICK,G.S.: Automated radiographic diagnosis via feature extraction and classification of cardiac size and shape descriptors. IEEE Trans.BME-19,1972,174.

KRUGER,R.P.;MAC GREGOR,C.B. and DARNDT,R.: Computer aided calculation of left ventricular cardiac volumes. In: Proc.6th.Hawai Int.Conf.Syst.Sci.1973,330.

KUERSCHNER,G.: Wirkung des Herzens auf die Blutbewegung. In: Handwörterbuch der Physiologie mit Rücksicht auf Physiologische Pathologie. Braunschweig,1844,16.

KUNDEL,H.L.;REVESZ,G.;ZISKIN,M.C. and SHEA,J.: The image and its influence on quantitative radiological data. Invest.Radiol.7,1972,187.

LANGE,P.E.;MOLDENHAUER,U.;STRAUME,K.;GILDBERG,P.;HUETTING,G. and HEINTZEN,P.H.: Analysis of the shape of the left and right ventricle by a special cast technique. Symp.Europ.Soc.Cardiol., Düsseldorf,15 March 1974.(Publ. in prep.).

LANTZ,B. and STRID,K.-G.: Contrast formation in fluoroscopic videodensitometry, part II. Acta Radiol.14,1973,406.

LARSSON,H. and KJELLBERG,S.R.: Roentgenological heart volume determination with special regard to pulse rate and position of the body. Acta Radiol.29,1948,159

LESHIN,S.J.;WILDENTHAL,K.;MULLINS,C.B. and MITCHELL,J.H.: Measurement of left ventricular dimensions from implanted radiopaque markers. J.Appl.Physiol.33, 1972,132.

LEVITSKY,S.;SCHUETTE,W.H.;KEMPNER,K.M.SLOANE,R.;SOUTHER,S.G.;MULLIN,E.M. and MORROW,A.G.: Experimental and early clinical evaluation of heart tracking (Radarkymography) as a noninvasive method for measuring myocardial contractility. Amer.J.Cardiol.32,1973,156.

LINDBERG,B.: Video kymography: an improved method for electrokymography. Thesis, Goeteborg,1972. (Tech.Rep. no 18).

LINDGREN,P.: Hemodynamic responses to contrast media. Invest.Radiol.5,1970,424.

LISSNER,J.: Der Wert der Modulationsübertragungsfunktion für die Beurteilung der Fernsehbildqualität. Fortschr.Roentgenstr.110,1968,87.

LOMAN,A. et COMANDON,J.: La radiocinematographie par la photographie des écrans renforsateurs. Bull.Mem.Soc.Radiol.Med.Paris,3,1911,127.

LUBBERTS,M.G. and ROSSMANN,K.: Modulation transfer function associated with geometrical unsharpness in medical radiography. Phys.Med.Biol.12,1967,65.

LUDBROOK,P.J.;KARLINER,J.S.;LONDON,A.;PETERSON,K.L.;LEOPOLD,G.R. and O'ROURKE, R.A.: Posterior wall velocity: an unreliable index of total left ventricular performance in patients with coronary artery disease. Amer.J.Cardiol.33,1974, 475.

LYSELL,G.;MARTENSON,B.K.A. and OMNELL,K.A.: Determination of small mass differences in roentgenography-I. Theoretical considerations. Acta Radiol.7,1968,42.

LYSHOLM,E.;NYLIN,G. and QUARNA,K.: The relation between the heart volume and stroke volume under physiological and pathological conditions. Acta Radiol.15, 1934,237.

MAC CORMICK,E.J.: Human factors engineering. New York,1970.

MAC DONALD,I.G.: The shape and movements of the human left ventricle during systole. Amer.J.Cardiol.26,1970,221.

MAC INTYRE,J.: X-ray records for the cinematograph. Arch.Skiagraphy,1,1897,37.

MARCUS,M.L.;SCHUETTE,W.H.;WHITEHOUSE,W.C.;BAILEY,J.J. and GLANCY,D.L.: An automated method for the measurement of ventricular volume. Circulation,45,1972,65

MARCUS,M.L.;SCHUETTE,W.H.;WHITEHOUSE,W.C.;BAILEY,J.J.;DOUGLAS,M.A. and GLANCY,D.I Use of a video system in the study of ventricular function in man. Amer.J. Cardiol.32,1973,175.

MEETEREN,A.VAN: Visual aspects of image intensification. Thesis, Utrecht,1973.

MEIJLER,F.L.;STRACKEE,J.;CAPELLE,F.J.L.VAN and PERRON,J.C.DU: Computer analysis of the RR-interval-contractility relationship during random stimulation of the isolated heart. Circulat.Res.22,1968,695.

MEIJLER,F.L.: The role of the heart in regulation of the circulation. Acta Physiol.Pharmacol.Neerl.15,1969,282.

MELLINK,J.H.: Roentgenfysische aspecten van het gebruik van kontrastmiddelen in de roentgendiagnostiek. J.Belge Radiol.44,1961,107.

MILLETT,D.C. and LARSON,I.W.: An easy way to analyse graphs. Hewlett-Packard J. June 1971,13.

MISTRETTA,C.A.;ORT,M.G.;CAMERON,J.R.;CRUMMY,A.B. and MORAN,P.R.: A multiple image subtraction technique for enhancing low contrast, periodic object. Invest. Radiol.8,1973,43.

MITCHELL,J.H. and MULLINS,C.B.: Dimensional analysis of left ventricular function In: Influencing myocardial contractility. Editors: R.D. Tanz,F. Kavaler and J. Roberts. New York,1967,117.

MITCHELL,J.H.;WILDENTHAL,K. and MULLINS,C.B.: Geometrical studies of the left ventricle utilizing biplane cinefluorography. Fed.Proc.28,1969,1334.

MOLDENHAUER,K.: Experimentelle Untersuchungen über die Schwachung Gepulster Röntgenstrahlung durch Kontrastmittel. Thesis, Kiel,1972.

MOLDENHAUER,K. und HEINTZEN,P.H.: Rechnergeneriertes raumliches Modell und Referenzsystem für den linken Ventrikel zur Untersuchung seines regionales Kontraktionsablaufes aus Angiokardiogrammen. In: Dig.3rd Yearly Conf. German.Biomed.Soc., Editors O. Anna and C. Hartwig, Hannover,15-17 May 1974,119.

MOND,H.;FENELON,T.;MAC DONALD,R. and SLOMAN,G.: Heart motion video tracking. Brit.Heart.J.35,1973,488.

MORGAN,R.H. and STURM,R.E.: The John Hopkins fluoroscopic screen intensifier. Radiology,57,1951,556.

MORITZ,F.: Eine Methode um beim Röntgenverfahren aus den Schattenbilde eines Gegenstandes dessern wahre Grösse zu Ermitteln und die exakte Bestimmung der Herzgrösze nach diesem Verfahren. Münch.Mediz.Wochenschr.47,1900,992.

194

MOSELEY,R.D. and RUST,J.H.: Diagnostic radiologic instrumentation. Editors: R.D. Moseley and J.H. Rust, Springfield,1965.

MOSELEY,R.D. and RUST,J.H.: Television in diagnostic radiology. Editors: R.D. Moseley and J.H. Rust, Birmingham,1969.

MUDD,J.G. and LOEFFEL,R.: A simple method for recording the ECG,PCG, or pressure tracing on the cineangiogram. Ire.Trans.Med.Electron.7,1960,228.

MULLINS,C.B.;LESHIN,S.J.;MIERZWIAK,D.S.;ALSOBROOK,H.D. and MITCHELL,J.H.: Changes in left ventricular function produced by the injection of contrast media. Amer.Heart J.83,1972,373.

N.C.R.H. Task force on X-ray image analysis and systems development, U.S.Dept. H.E.W.: Obtaining the maximum benefit of radiation exposure in diagnostic radiology through improved production and utilization of image information. Rep. Pb. 184130,1968,1.

NELSON,C.N. and LIPCHIK,E.O.: A computer method for calculation of left ventricular volume from biplane angiocardiograms. Invest.Radiol.1,1966,139.

NOBLE,M.I.M.;MILNE,E.N.C.;GOERKE,R.J.;CARLSSON,E.;DOMENECH,R.J.;SAUNDERS,K.B. and HOFFMAN,J.I.E.: Left ventricular filling and diastolic pressure-volume relations in the conscious dog. Circul.Res.24,1969(a),269.

NOBLE,M.I.M.;WYLER,J.;MILNE,E.N.C.;TRENCHARD,D. and GUZ,A.: Effect of changes in heart rate on left ventricular performance in conscious dogs. Circul.Res.24, 1969(b),285.

NOBLE,M.I.M.: Problems in the definition of contractility in terms of myocardial mechanics. Europ.J.Cardiol.1,1973,209.

OLIN,T.: Studies in angiographic technique. Thesis, Lund,1963.

OOSTERKAMP,W.J.: Monochromatic X-rays for medical fluoroscopy and radiography. Medica Mundi,7,1961(a),68.

OOSTERKAMP,W.J. und SCHUT,TH.G.: Magnetische Speicherung von Röntgenbilder. Elektromedizin,6,1961(b),147.

OSYPKA,P.: The television monitor-a multipurpose medical data display. In: Visual display of biomedical data. Int.Fed.Med.Biol.Engng.Publ.M-5, Melbourne, 1971(a),7.

OSYPKA,P.: New techniques for processing medical videosignals and handling of reference data on videodisk recording. In: Roentgen-,cine- and videodensitometry. Editor: P.H. Heintzen, Stuttgart,1971(b),61.

PALMIERI,G.G.: Sulla possibilita di ricostruire il coure in plastica dal vivente con il sussido dei raggi X. Malat.Coure,4,1920,69. (Quoted in: Carlsson,1970).

PALMIERI,G.G.: Uber meine Methode der plastischen Darstellung des Herzens am Lebenden. ("Radioplastik"). Acta Radiol. Stockholm,10,1929,127.

PENN,WH.H.A.M.: Pulstechniek en snelcinematografie in de Röntgendiagnostiek. Thesis, Utrecht,1967.

PERKINS,W.J.: The functions of display systems in biomedical research. In: Visual display of biomedical data. Int.Fed.Med.Biol.Engng.Publ.M-5, Melbourne, 1971,1.

PETERSON,K.L.;SKLOVEN,D.;LUDBROOK,PH.;UTHER,J.B. and ROSS.J.: Comparison of isovolumic and ejection phase indices of myocardial performance in man. Circulation,49,1974,1088.

PFEILER,M.: Lineaire Systeme zur Ubertragung zeitabhängiger Ortsfunktionen und Bilder. Nachr.T.Zeitschr.2,1968,97.

PHARMACHEMIE,N.V.: Isopaque metrizoaat, een intravasculair contrastmiddel voor de angiografie en de urografie. Haarlem,1968,1-44.

PIKE,W.S.: Some television image enhancement techniques. Ann.N.Y.Acad.Sci.97, 1962,395.

PILZ,F. und SCHAEFFER,H.: Fotoelektrischer Zeitgestab für Fernsehbilder. Radio-Mentor,12,1964,938.

POLDER,L.J.VAN DER: Targetstabilization effects in television pick-up tubes. Philips Res.Rep.22,1967,178.

PORSTMANN,W.;GEISSLER,W. und BURGEMEISTER,G.: Die percutane Katheterisierung der vier Herzhöhlen. Fortschr.Röntgenstr.97,1962,449.

RACKLEY,C.E. and HOOD,W.P.: Derivation of cardiac mechanical parameters from serial biplane angiocardiograms. J.Appl.Physiol.$\underline{24}$,1968,254.

RAO,U.V.G. and BATES,L.M.: The modulation transfer functions of X-ray focal spots. Phys.Med.Biol.$\underline{14}$,1968,93.

RAO,U.V.G.;CLARK,R.L. and GAYLER,B.W.: Radiographic magnification: a critical, theoretical and practical analysis. Appl.Radiol.1,1973,37.

RAPHAEL,M.J. and ALLWORK,S.P.: Angiographic anatomy of the left ventricle. Clin. Radiol.$\underline{25}$,1974,95.

RECOURT,A.: Allgemeine Trends in der Röntgendiagnostik. Röntgen-Bl.$\underline{25}$,1972,145.

REDLER,U. und BUEHLMEYER,K.: Herzkatheterisierung mit fortlaufender Protokoll Herstellung durch einen Digitaldrucker. Electromedica,$\underline{5}$,1972,185.

REDMAN,J.D.;WOLTON,W.P. and SHUTTLEWORTH,E.: Use of holography to make truly three-dimensional X-ray images. Nature,220,1968,58.

REINSCH,CH.: Smoothing by spline functions. Numer.Math.$\underline{10}$,1967,177.

REITSMA,H. und LUITEN.A.L.: Automatische Herzrandbestimmung und Planimetrie mit Hilfe der Videodensitonetrie. In: Densitometrie in der Radiologie. Editor: F. Heuck, Stuttgart,1973,128.

REVESZ,G.;KUNDEL,H. and HAAS,C.: Electronic techniques for radiological image processing. Med.Biol.Engng,$\underline{7}$,1969,393.

RICE,R.P. and BARNHARDT,L.E.: A simplified subtraction technique. Amer.J.Roentgenol.$\underline{97}$,1966,529.

RITMAN,E.L.;STURM,E. and WOOD,E.H.: A biplane roentgenvideometry system for dynamic (60/sec) studies of the shape and size of circulation structures, particulary the left ventricle. In: Roentgen-,cine- and videodensitometry. Editor: P.H. Heintzen, Stuttgart,1971,179.

RITMAN,E.L.;JOHNSON,A.J.;STURM,R.E. and WOOD,E.H.: The television camera in dynamic videoangiography. Radiology,$\underline{107}$,1973,417.

ROBB,R.A.: Computer-aided contour determination and dynamic display of individual cardiac chambers from digitized serial angiocardiographic film. In: Roentgen-, cine- and videodensitometry. Editor: P.H. Heintzen, Stuttgart,1971,170.

ROBB,R.A.;GREENLEAF,J.F.;RITMAN,E.L.;JOHNSON,S.A.;SJOSTRAND,J.D.;HERMAN,G.T. and WOOD,E.H.: Three-dimensional visualization of the intact thorax and contents: a technique for cross-sectional reconstruction from multiplanar X-ray views. Comput.Biomed.Res.$\underline{7}$,1974,395.

ROBIN,CH.: Notes historiques sur la capacité absolue et relative des cavités du coeur. J.Anat.Physiol.Norm.Path. Paris,$\underline{1}$,1864,420.

ROCKOFF,S.D.: Techniques of data extraction from radiological images. Invest. Radiol.$\underline{7}$,1972,206.

ROEHLER,R.H.A.: The visibility of structures in the presence of optical noise and its dependence on noise spectrum, presentation time and repetition frequency. In: Television in diagnostic radiology. Editors: R.D. Moseley and J.H. Rust, Birmingham,1969,357.

ROENTGEN,C.W.: Uber eine neue Art von Strahlen. Sitzungsberichte der Physikalisch Medizinischen Gesellschaft, Würzberg,1895,132.

ROHRER,F.: Volumenbestimmung von Dörperhöhlen und Organen auf orthodiagraphischen Weg. Fortschr.Röntgenschr.24,1916,285.

ROSENFELD,A. and THURSTON,M.: Edge and curve detection for visual scene analysis. Rept.Af CRL-70-0488/CSC Tech.Rept.70-128,1970.

ROSS,J.;SONNENBLICK,E.H.;COVELL,J.W.;KAISER,G.A. and SPIRO,D.: The architecture of the heart in systole and diastole-technique of rapid fixation and analysis of left ventricular geometry. Circul.Res.$\underline{21}$,1967,409.

ROSSMANN,K.: A method for measuring one-dimensional spatial frequency spectra of objects in medical radiology. In: Television in diagnostic radiology. Editors: R.D. Moseley and J.H. Rust, Birmingham,1969(a),412.

ROSSMANN,K.: Point spread-function, line spread-function and modulation transfer function. Radiology,$\underline{93}$,1969(b),257.

ROTH,W. and STRICKHOLM,G.: Subtraction radiology by electro-optical means. Invest.Radiol.$\underline{5}$,1970,164.

ROY,H. and ADAMI,C.G.: Remarks on the failure of the heart from overstrain. Brit.Med.J.$\underline{2}$,1888,1321.

RUGGELS,H.E.: X-ray motion pictures of the thorax. Radiology,$\underline{5}$,1925,44.

RUSHMER,R.F. and CRYSTAL,D.K.: Changes in configuration of the ventricular chambers during the cardiac cycle. Circulation,$\underline{4}$,1951(a),211.

RUSHMER,R.F. and THAL,N.: The mechanics of ventricular contraction- a cinefluorographic study. Circulation,4,1951(b),219.

RUSHMER,R.F.;CRYSTAL,D.K. and WAGNER,C.: The functional anatomy of ventricular contraction. Circul.Res.$\underline{1}$,1953,162.

RUSHMER,R.F.;FINLAYSON,B.L. and NASH,A.A.: Shrinkage of the heart in anesthetized thoracotomized dogs. Circul.Res.$\underline{2}$,1954,22.

RUTISHAUSER,W.: Kreislaufanalyse mittels Röntgendensitometrie. Bern,1969.(170 refs).

SALVESEN,S.;NILSEN,P.L. and HOLTERMAN,H.: Effects of calcium and magnesium ions on the systemic and local toxicities of the N-methyl glucamine (meglumine) salt of metriozoic acid (metrazoate). Acta Radiol.Supp.$\underline{270}$,1966,180.

SANDLER,H. and DODGE,H.T.: The use of single plane angiocardiograms for the calculation of left ventricular volume in man. Amer.Heart J.$\underline{75}$,1968,325.

SANDLER,H. and GHISTA,D.N.: Mechanical and dynamic implication of dimensional measurements of the left ventricle. Fed.Proc.$\underline{28}$,1969,1344.

SANDLER,H.: Dimensional analysis of the heart. Amer.J.Med.Sci.$\underline{26}$,1970,56. (159 refs).

SANDLER,H. and RASMUSSEN,D.: Angiographic analysis of heart geometry. In: Roentgen-,cine- and videodensitometry. Editor: P.H. Heintzen, Stuttgart,1971,212.

SANDLER,H.: Left ventricular volume, mass and related measures; usefulness in determination of ventricular function. In: Quantitation in cardiology. Editors H.A. Snellen;H.C. Hemker;P.G. Hugenholtz and J.H. van Bemmel, Leiden,1972,189.

SANDLER,H. and ALDERMAN,E.: Determination of left ventricular size and shape. Circul-Res.$\underline{34}$,1974,1.

SANMARCO,M.E. and BARTLE,S.H.: Measurement of left ventricular volume in the canine heart by biplane angiocardiography: accuracy of the method using different model analogies. Circul.Res.$\underline{19}$,1966,11.

SANTAMORE,W.P.;MEO,F.N.DI and LYNCH,P.R.: A comparative study of various single-plane cineangiographic methods to measure left-ventricular volume. IEEE Trans.BME-$\underline{20}$,1973,417.

SARNOFF,S.J.;MITCHELL,J.H.;GILMORE,J.P. and REMENSNYDER,J.P.: Homeometric autoregulation in the heart. Circul.Res.$\underline{8}$,1960,1077.

SARNOFF,S.J. and MITCHELL,J.H.: The control of the function of the heart. In: Handbook of Physiology,Vol.$\underline{1}$,sect.2,489, Washington,1962.

SAYANAGI,K.: Consideration of non-linearity in image-transfer systems. In: Television in diagnostic radiology. Editors: R.D. Moseley and J.H. Rust, Birmingham,1969,399.

SCHAD,N.: Die intermittierende Kontrastmittelinjektion in das Herz. Stuttgart, 1967.SCHEFFE,H.: The analysis of variance, New York,1959.

SCHELBERT,H.R.;KREUZER,H.;DITTRICH,J.;REITSMA,H. und SPILLER,P.: Videometrische Ventrikelflächenbestimmung mit halbautomatischer Korrektur des Bildhintergrundes. Res.Exp.Med. Berlin,$\underline{148}$,1972,66.

SCHMIEL,F.K.;SCHELBERT,H.R.;DITTRICH,J. and KREUZER,H.: Detection of abnormal LV-wall motion and altered local myocardial function by means of a new, automated method. In: VI Congreso Europeo de Cardiologia, Madrid,1972.

SCHBER,H.: Allgemeine physiologische Grundregeln für die Detailwahrnehmung in Röntgenbild. In: Bildgüte in der Radiologie. Editor: F.-E Stieve, Stuttgart, 1966,122.

SCHOHL,H.H.: Röntgenvideometrische Bestimmung von Modellvolumina als Grundlage eines Verfahrens zur automatischen Messung des Herzkammervolumes. Thesis, Kiel,1972.

SCHOKNECHT,G.: Quantitative Beschreibung von Kontrastmittelaufnahmen. In: Bildgüte in der Radiologie. Editor: F.-E. Stieve, Stuttgart,1966,268.

SCHOTT,O.: Bildqualität und Strahlendosisprobleme in der Röntgendiagnostik. Röntgen-bl.14,1961,1.
SCHOTT,O.: Die Modulationsübertragungsfunktion in der Radiologie. In: Bildgüte in der Radiologie. Editor: F.-E. Stieve, Stuttgart,1966,268.
SCHOTT,O.: The X-ray pattern and its properties. In: Television in diagnostic radiology. Editors: R.D. Moseley and J.H. Rust, Birmingham,1969,141.
SEEMAN,H.E.: Physical and photographic principles of medical radiography. New York,1968.
SIMON,A.L.;SCHUETTE,S.A.L. and WHITEHOUSE,W.C.: Television planimetry. Radiology,94,1970,203.
SINCLAIR,J.D.;SUTTERER,W.F.;WOLFORD,J.L.;ARMELIN,E. and WOOD,E.H.: Problems in comparison of dye-dilution curves with densitometric variations at the same site in the circulation measured from simultaneous cineangiograms. Mayo Clin.Proc.35,1960,764.
SOLOFF,L.A.: On measuring left ventricle volume. Amer.J.Cardiol.18,1966,2.
SONNENBLICK,E.H.: Contractility in the intact heart: progress and problems. Europ.J.Cardiol.1,1974,319.
SOUTHWORTH,G.R.: A magnetic disk video scan converter. J.Soc.Mot.Pict.Telev. Engrs.77,1968,624.
SPIEGLER,G.: Physikalische Grundlagen der Röntgendiagnostik. Stuttgart,1957.
STARLING,E.H.: The Linacre lecture on the law of the heart. London,1918.
STEIGER,U.;HARLANDER,W.;DELUIGI,B.;OSYPKA,P. and RUTISHAUSER,W.: Application of television technics for data monitoring and processing in cardiology and radiology. Dig.10th.Int.Conf.Med.Biol.Engng. Dresden,13-17 Aug.1973,sess.36-2.
STEWART,G.H.: High rate physiological dynamics in three-dimensional space: their acquisition via cineradiography. Thesis, Philadelphia,1968.
STEWART,G.H.;LYNCH,P.R. and GIMENEZ,J.L.: Versatile techniques for the analysis of multodimensional information. Med.Biol.Engng.7,1969,435.
STIEVE,F.-E.: Bildgüte in der Radiologie. Editor: F.-E. Stieve, Stuttgart,1966(a).
STIEVE,F.-E.: Kontrast und Schärfe im Röntgenbild der Lunge. In: Bildgüte in der Radiologie. Editor: F.-E. Stieve, Stuttgart,1966(b),217.
STIMSON,M.J.;JANZ,R.F. and GOTT,A.H.: Current status of densitometric left ventricular volume computation. In: Proc.S.P.I.E.Seminar.Quant.Imagery in the Bio-Med.Sciences. Editor: R.E. Herron, Houston,10-12 May,1971,23.
STRACKEE,J.;HOELEN,A.J.;ZIMMERMAN,A.N.E. and MEIJLER,F.L.: Artificial atrial fibrillation: an artifact? Circul.Res.28,1971,441.
STRID,K.-G. and LANTZ,B.: Contrast formation in fluoroscopic videodensitometry. Acta Radiol.14,1973,395.
STURM,R.E. and WOOD,E.H.: The video quantizer: an electronic photometer to measure contrast in roentgenfluoroscopic images. Mayo Clin.Proc.43,1968,803.
STURM,R.E.;RITMAN,E.L.;HANSEN,R.J. and WOOD,E.H.: Recording of multichannel analog data and video images on the same video tape or disk. J.Appl.Physiol.36, 1974,761.
SUGA,H. and SAGAWA,K.: Instantaneous pressure-volume relationships and their ratio in the excised, supported canine left ventricle. Circul.Res.35,1974,117.
SUSMAN,N. and DIBOLL,W.B.: Fluid dynamics in the tip of the multiholed angiographic catheter. Radiology,92,1969,843.
TAKAHASHI,S and SHINOZAKI,T.: Solidography of the heart. Acta Radiol. Stockholm, 41,1954,435.
TAKENAKA,E.;KINOSHITA,K. and NAKAJIMA,R.: Modulation transfer function of the intensity distribution of the roentgen focal spot. Acta Radiol.7,1968,263.
TEMPLES,J.T. and KENT,K.M.: On-line computation of stroke volume from aortic flow Med.Res.Engng.8,1969,27.
TEVES,M.C. en TOL,T.: Electronische versterking van röntgenbeelden. Philips, Techn.Tijdschr.14,1952,65.
THOMPSON,B.J.: The dilemma of image quality. In: Proc.Electro-Optical Systems Design Conf. New York City,22-24 Sep.1970,3.
TIMM,C.: Die Blutbewegung in der Aorta. Röntgenkinematographische Untersuchung mit Zeitdehnung an Hunden und Katzen. Pflügers Arch.Ges.Physiol.249,1947,261.

TIMMER,F.: Evaluation of X-ray imaging systems in terms of transfer functions. Paper IEE/IERE meeting on X-ray image intensifier systems, London,14 June, 1973. (publ.Image Quality Group, Philips Medical Systems Division, Eindhoven).

TRENHOLM,B.G.;WINTER,D.A.;MYMIN,D. and LANSDOWN,E.L.: Computer determination of left ventricular volume using videodensitometry. Med.Biol.Engng.$\underline{10}$,1972,163.

TRENHOLM,B.G.;WINTER,D.A.;BEIMER,G.D.;MYMIN,D.;LANSDOWN,E.L. and SHARMA,G.P.: Automated ventricular volume calculations from single plane images. Radiology,$\underline{112}$,1974,299.

UNGERLEIDER,H.E. and CLARK,C.P.: A study of the transverse diameter of the heart silhouette with prediction table based on the teleoroentgenogram. Amer.Heart J. 1 $\underline{17}$,1939,92.

VENEMA,H.W. and OVERWEG,J.: Analysis of the size and shape of cross-sections of muscular fibers. Med.Biol.Engng.$\underline{12}$,1974,681.

VLASSENROOT,G.E.: The subtraction method in miniature film angiocardiography. Thesis, Amsterdam,1961.

VOGEL,G.W.: Möglichkeiten und Fehler einer automatisierten Volumenbestimmung aus Röntgenfernsehsignalen an Modellen. Thesis, Kiel,1971.

WACHSMANN,F. und DIMOTSIS,A.: Kurven und Tabelle für die Strahlentherapie. Stuttgart,1957.

WERF,T.VAN DER: Directe en indirecte stroommeting in het hart en de grote bloedvaten. Thesis, Groningen,1965.

WHITE,G.: Video recording, record and replay systems. London,1972.

WHITHAM,G.E.: The determination of display screen size and resolution based on perceptual and information limitations. In: Proc.3rd Nat.Symp. on Inf.Display, San Diego,Feb.1964,104.

WILDENTHAL,K. and MITCHELL,J.H.: Dimensional analysis of the left ventricle in unanaesthesized dogs. J.Appl.Physiol.$\underline{27}$,1969,112.

WINTER,D.A. and REIMER,G.D.: Quantization errors in calculation of volumes areas and coordinates in medical images. In: Proc.S.P.I.E.$\underline{32}$,1972,107.

WISCOMB,W.K.: A hardware system for man-machine interaction in the study of left ventricular dynamics. In: Roentgen-,cine and videodensitometry. Editor: P.H. Heintzen, Stuttgart,1971,165.

WISE,R.E. and GANSON,J.: Subtraction technic: video-and colour methods. Radiology,$\underline{86}$,1966,814.

WOLSCHENDORF,$\overline{K}$. und VANSELOV,K.: Uber die Charakterisierung der Strahlenqualität weicher Röntgenstrahlen durch effektive Wellenlänge bei densitometrischen Meszverfahren. Biomediz.Techn.$\underline{18}$,1973,230.

WOOD,E.H.: Speculations concerning present and future developments in indicator-dilution technics. Circul.Res.$\underline{10}$,1962,569.

WOOD,E.H.;STURM,R.E. and SANDERS,$\overline{J}$.J.: Data processing in cardiovascular physiology with particular reference to roentgenvideodensitometry. Mayo Clin.Proc. $\underline{39}$,1964,849.

WOOD,E.H.;RITMAN,E.L.;STURM,R.E.;JOHNSON,S.;SPIVAK,P.L.;GILBERT,B.K. and SMITH,H.C.: The problem of determination of the roentgendensity. Dimensions and shape of homogeneous objects from biplane roentgenographic data with particular reference to angiography. In: Proc.10th Ann. San Diego Biomed.Symp.$\underline{11}$, 1972,3.

WIJK VAN BRIEVINGH,R.P.VAN: Quantitative videoangiocardiography, a method for measuring the heart's pumping function. Delft Progr.Rep. Series B,$\underline{1}$,1973(a),11.

WIJK VAN BRIEVINGH,R.P.VAN;RICHTERING BLENKEN,A.;SNEEK,J.H.J. and ZIMMERMAN, A.N.E.: Subtraction as a tool in quantitative videoangiocardiography. Dig.10th Conf.Med.Biol.Engng. Dresden,13-17Aug.1973(b),Sess.6-5.

WIJK VAN BRIEVINGH,R.P.VAN;RICHTERING BLENKEN,A.;POELGEEST,R.VAN;SNEEK,J.H.J.; WERF,T.VAN DER;ZIMMERMAN,A.N.E. and MEIJLER,F.L.: A measurement system for left ventricular volume determination. Europ.J.Cardiol.$\underline{1}$,1974(a),259.

WIJK VAN BRIEVINGH,R.P.VAN;HEMELAAR,A.;COENEN,A.J.R.M.;KRIJGER,T.J.C.DE;POELGEEST R.VAN and SNEEK,J.H.J.: Integrated information recording during angiocardiography. In: Dig.Europ.Conf.Electronics"EUROCON'74", Amsterdam,22-26 April 1974 (b),Sess.E-2-6.

WIJK VAN BRIEVINGH,R.P.VAN and HEETHAAR,J.: Computer development of the three-dimensional geometry of the left ventricle and calculations of left ventricular volume. In: Cardiovascular physics of medical procedures and devices. Editors: D.N. Ghista;E. van Vollenhoven and W.J. Yang. Vol.III Diagnostics, Part I, Cardiac contractility, Chapter 4. Delft,1975 (accepted for publication 26 Nov. 1974).

YANG,S.S.;BENTIVOGLIO,L.G.;MARANHAO,V. and GOLDBERG,H.: From cardiac catheterization data to hemodynamic parameters. Philadelphia,1972.

YIN,F.C.P. and TOMPKINS,W.R.; A video dimension analyser. IEEE Trans.BME-$\underline{19}$,1972, 376.

ZAHN,C.T. and ROSKIES,R.Z.: Fourier descriptors for plane closed curves. IEEE Trans.Comput.C-$\underline{21}$,1972,269.

ZAR,J.H.: Biostatistical analysis. Englewood Cliffs,N.J.1974.

ZIEDSES DES PLANTES,B.: Planigraphie en subtractie. Thesis, Utrecht,1934.

ZIEDSES DES PLANTES,B.: Subtraktion. Stuttgart,1961.

ZIEDSES DES PLANTES,B.: Die Bildgüte bei der Subtraktion. In: Bildgüte in der Radiologie. Editor: F.-E. Stieve, Stuttgart,1966,278.

ZIMMERMANN,R. und BUSSMANN,W.-D.: Kombinierte TV-Monitor-Datensichtstation zur Aufzeichnung und Auswertung von Videobildern. Biomediz.Techn.$\underline{16}$,1971,189.

ZIMMERMANN,R.;AMELING,W.;BUSSMANN,W.-D. and EFFERT,S.: Visual display unit for biplane roentgen-videometry with simultaneous analog data presentation. Med.Biol.Engng.$\underline{10}$,1972,784.

ZIMMERMANN,R.;BUSSMANN,W.-D.;SCHMIDT,M.;AMELING,W. und EFFERT,S.: Röntgenvideo-densitometrische Verfahren zur Ventrikelvolumenbestimmung unter Verwendung eines Video-lichtgriffels und digitalen Konturspeicher. Biomediz.Techn.$\underline{18}$, 1973,124.

ZISKIN,M.C.;REVESZ,G.;KUNDEL,H.L. and SHEA,F.J.: Spatial frequency spectra of radiographic images. Radiology,$\underline{98}$,1971,507.

200

2. *List of Internal Reports*

SNEEK,J.H.J. (MScEE.-thesis): "Tijdprogrammering voor gefractioneerde röntgen-contraststofinjectie t.b.v. linkerhartkamervolumebepaling." Internal Report Medical Engineering Group,M82,1971.

HOEKSTRA,A. (MScEE.-thesis): "Het aangeven van een contour in een röntgentelevisiebeeld met een lichtpen/scan converter kombinatie." Internal Report Medical Engineering Group,M88,1971.

HEMELAAR,A. (MScEE.-thesis): "VIDICOR, een apparaat voor retrospektief-momentane videopresentatie van analoge signalen." Internal Report Medical Engineering Group,M89,1972.

BERG,J.G. VAN DEN .en GRAAF,H. VAN DER: "Het bepalen van het eindsystolisch moment van de hartslag uit ECG,P_v en P_a." Internal Report Medical Engineering Group,M91,1972.

COENEN,A.J.R.M:"Een video-computer interface voor bepaling van het linkerhartkamervolume". Internal Report Medical Engineering Group,M92,1972.

COENEN,A.J.R.M.:"ANACOR,(Analoog-video omzetter)". Internal Report Medical Engineering Group,M101,1973.

PADT,A.VAN DER:"Het koderen van videobanden met signalen op het audiospoor ten behoeve van een geautomatiseerde 'tape-o-theek'". Internal Report Medical Engineering Group,M104,1973.

KRIJGER,T.C.J.DE,(MScEE-thesis):"DIGICOR,een apparaat,waarmee digitale informatie wordt gecodeerd op de 32 eerste en laatste 32 lijnen van een TV-raster". Internal Report Laboratory for Switching Techniques and Data Processing, 051560-28,1973,22.

VEEN,B.L.J.VAN,:"Een digitaal contourgeheugen,annex Video Computer Interface". Internal Report Medical Engineering Group,M107,1974.

SILVA,M.J.DA,:"Smoothing en plotting procedures voor meetresultaten van quantitatieve videoangiocardiografie". Internal Report Medical Engineering Group, M116,1974.

VULKER,J.H.J.M.(MSc.-thesis in Industrial Design Engineering):"Ergonomische factoren,van invloed op het MMS-blok in de meetopstelling voor kwantitatieve videoangiocardiografie". Internal Report Department of Industrial Design Engineering and Centre for Medical Engineering,1975.

FRANSEN,A.A.J. en SPOELSTRA,A.W.M.:"Het meten van de temporele en spatiële modulatieoverdrachtsfuncties van een tweevlaks röntgeninstallatie". Internal Report Medical Engineering Group,M121,1975.

ACKNOWLEDGEMENTS

The typework of the manuscript in several phases has been in the able
hands of Mrs. Hanneke Wentholt-Eggels and Miss Kitty Schoute.
The figures have been prepared in the technical illustration department
by W.T.J. van Kan an J. Keuvelaar and by the photographers J.C. van der
Krogt, P.A. Beijlsmit, H.F. Breuker and P. de Meijer. J.M. Brans has
contributed an important part as a dedicated literature retriever;
Mrs D.J. Weisz-van Limburgh has been a great help in aquiring the
publications selected and in correcting the list of references. In the
Computer Group Cardiology, R. van Poelgeest, J. Heethaar and G. Rol
have dealt with many software problems; the discussions with A.J. Hoelen
in the initial stage have proved very inspiring. The timing system for
using the X-ray installation as a measurement tool has been realized
by the devoted work of J.H.J. Sneek. A. Richtering Blenken has developed essential hardware with great ingenuity. I. van Egmond, C.J.
Verleg and J. Rikken have given invaluable assistance in the construction of prototypes. The ventricular casts have been prepared by E. van
Dam. The advice on ergonomic problems given by J.H.J.M. Vulker has
filled gaps which otherwise would have been pitfalls.
I am grateful to dr. W. Herstel and dr. H.R. Marcuse for many discussions
and to G.R. van den Broek for correcting the English text. The smooth
contacts with the publisher have facilitated the realization of this
publication.